Treatment of Mutilating Hand Injuries: An International Perspective

Editor

S. RAJA SABAPATHY

HAND CLINICS

www.hand.theclinics.com

Consulting Editor
KEVIN C. CHUNG

November 2016 • Volume 32 • Number 4

ELSEVIER

1600 John F. Kennedy Boulevard • Suite 1800 • Philadelphia, Pennsylvania, 19103-2899

http://www.theclinics.com

HAND CLINICS Volume 32, Number 4
November 2016 ISSN 0749-0712, ISBN-13: 978-0-323-47684-3

Editor: Jennifer Flynn-Briggs
Developmental Editor: Kristen Helm

Hand Clinics (ISSN 0749-0712) is published quarterly by Elsevier Inc., 360 Park Avenue South, New York, NY 10010-1710. Months of publication are February, May, August, and November. Business and Editorial Offices: 1600 John F. Kennedy Blvd., Ste. 1800, Philadelphia, PA 19103-2899. Customer Service Office: 3251 Riverport Lane, Maryland Heights, MO 63043. Periodicals postage paid at New York, NY and at additional mailing offices. Subscription price is $390.00 per year (domestic individuals), $687.00 per year (domestic institutions), $100.00 per year (domestic students/residents), $445.00 per year (Canadian individuals), $799.00 per year (Canadian institutions), $530.00 per year (international individuals), $799.00 per year (international institutions), and $256.00 per year (international and Canadian students/residents). Foreign air speed delivery is included in all *Clinics* subscription prices. All prices are subject to change without notice. **POSTMASTER:** Send address changes to *Hand Clinics*, Elsevier Health Sciences Division, Subscription Customer Service, 3251 Riverport Lane, Maryland Heights, MO 63043. Customer Service (orders, claims, online, change of address): Elsevier Health Sciences Division, Subscription **Customer Service, 3251 Riverport Lane, Maryland Heights, MO 63043. Tel: 1-800-654-2452 (U.S. and Canada); 314-447-8871 (outside U.S. and Canada). Fax: 314-447-8029. E-mail: journalscustomerservice-usa@elsevier.com (for print support); journalsonlinesupport-usa@elsevier.com (for online support).**

Reprints. For copies of 100 or more of articles in this publication, please contact the Commercial Reprints Department, Elsevier Inc., 360 Park Avenue South, New York, New York 10010-1710. Tel.: 212-633-3874; Fax: 212-633-3820; E-mail: reprints@elsevier.com.

Hand Clinics is covered in *MEDLINE/PubMed (Index Medicus), Current Contents/Clinical Medicine, EMBASE/Excerpta Medica,* and *ISI/BIOMED.*

Contributors

CONSULTING EDITOR

KEVIN C. CHUNG, MD, MS
Charles B.G. de Nancrede Professor of
Surgery; Professor of Plastic Surgery and
Orthopaedic Surgery; Chief of Hand Surgery,
Section of Plastic Surgery, Department of
Surgery, University of Michigan Health System;
Assistant Dean for Faculty Affairs, Associate
Director of Global REACH, University of
Michigan Medical School, Ann Arbor, Michigan

EDITOR

**S. RAJA SABAPATHY, MS (Gen), MCh
(Plastic), DNB (Plastic), FRCS (Edin),
MAMS**
Chairman, Division of Plastic Surgery, Hand
Surgery, Reconstructive Microsurgery and
Burns, Ganga Hospital, Coimbatore,
Tamil Nadu, India

AUTHORS

NIDAL FARHAN ALDEEK, MD, MSc
Department of Plastic and Reconstructive
Surgery, Chang Gung Memorial Hospital,
Chang Gung Medical College, Chang Gung
University, Taipei, Taiwan

HEATHER L. BALTZER, MSc, MD, FRCS(C)
Toronto Western Hand Program, University
Health Network; Assistant Professor,
University of Toronto, Toronto, Ontario,
Canada

**PRAVEEN BHARDWAJ, MS (Ortho), DNB
(Ortho), FNB (Hand & Microsurgery), EDHS**
Consultant, Hand & Wrist Surgery and
Reconstructive Microsurgery, Ganga Hospital,
Coimbatore, Tamil Nadu, India

KEVIN C. CHUNG, MD, MS
Charles B.G. de Nancrede Professor of
Surgery; Professor of Plastic Surgery and
Orthopaedic Surgery; Chief of Hand Surgery,
Section of Plastic Surgery, Department of
Surgery, University of Michigan Health System;
Assistant Dean for Faculty Affairs, Associate
Director of Global REACH, University of
Michigan Medical School, Ann Arbor, Michigan

FRANCISCO DEL PIÑAL, MD, Dr Med
Private Practice, Instituto de Cirugía
Plástica y de la Mano, Hospital La Luz, Madrid,
Spain; Instituto de Cirugía Plástica y de la
Mano, Hospital Mutua Montañesa, Santander,
Spain

DAVID ELLIOT, MA, BM BCh, FRCS
Consultant, Department of Plastic Surgery,
St Andrews Centre for Plastic Surgery & Burns,
Chelmsford, Essex, United Kingdom

ANTHONY FOO, MD
Department of Hand & Reconstructive
Microsurgery, National University Health
System, Singapore, Singapore

AVIRAM M. GILADI, MD, MS
Resident, Section of Plastic Surgery,
Department of Surgery, University of Michigan
Health System, Ann Arbor, Michigan

DAVID GRAHAM, BPhty(hons), MBBS, FRACS(Orth), FAOrthA
Hand Surgeon, Department of Plastic, Hand &
Reconstructive Microsurgery and Burns,
Ganga Hospital, Coimbatore, Tamil Nadu,
India

LEENA JAIN, MS, MCh (Plastic Surgery)
Consultant Plastic Surgeon, Fortis Raheja
Hospital, Mumbai, India

JINSOO KIM, MD
Department of Plastic and Reconstructive
Surgery, Gwang-Myeong Sung-Ae General
Hospital, Gwangmyeong, Gyungki-do,
Korea

SAMIR M. KUMTA, MS, MCh (Plastic Surgery)
Consultant Plastic Surgeon, Lilavati Hospital
and Research Centre, Bandra Reclamation,
Mumbai, India

DONGCHUL LEE, MD
Department of Plastic and Reconstructive
Surgery, Gwang-Myeong Sung-Ae General
Hospital, Gwangmyeong, Gyungki-do, Korea

KYUNGJIN LEE, MD
Department of Plastic and Reconstructive
Surgery, Gwang-Myeong Sung-Ae General
Hospital, Gwangmyeong, Gyungki-do, Korea

YU-TE LIN, MD
Department of Plastic and Reconstructive
Surgery, Chang Gung Memorial Hospital,
Chang Gung Medical College, Chang Gung
University, Taipei, Taiwan

STEVEN L. MORAN, MD
Professor, Division of Orthopedic Surgery,
Department of Hand Surgery; Departmental
Chair; Professor, Division of Plastic Surgery,
Mayo Clinic, Rochester, Minnesota

RAJENDRA NEHETE, MS, MCh, DNB (Plastic Surgery)
Consultant Plastic, Hand and Microvascular
Surgeon, Vedant Hospital, Nashik, India

DAVIDE PENNAZZATO, MD
Clinical Fellow, Orthopaedics and
Traumatology, Department of Biotechnology
and Life Sciences (DBSV), University of
Insubria, Varese, Italy

KAVITHA RANGANATHAN, MD
Resident, Section of Plastic Surgery,
Department of Surgery, University of Michigan
Health System, Ann Arbor, Michigan

SIYOUNG ROH, MD
Department of Plastic and Reconstructive
Surgery, Gwang-Myeong Sung-Ae General
Hospital, Gwangmyeong, Gyungki-do,
Korea

S. RAJA SABAPATHY, MS (Gen), MCh (Plastic), DNB (Plastic), FRCS (Edin), MAMS
Chairman, Division of Plastic Surgery, Hand
Surgery, Reconstructive Microsurgery and
Burns, Ganga Hospital, Coimbatore,
Tamil Nadu, India

AJEESH SANKARAN, MS (Ortho)
Registrar, Department of Plastic, Hand &
Reconstructive Microsurgery and Burns,
Ganga Hospital, Coimbatore, Tamil Nadu,
India

SANDEEP J. SEBASTIN, MD
Department of Hand & Reconstructive
Microsurgery, National University Health
System, Singapore, Singapore

SUNIL M. THIRKANNAD, MD
Clinical Associate Professor of Hand Surgery
(Gen. Surg) & Clinical Associate Professor of
Orthopedic Surgery; Christine M. Kleinert
Institute for Hand & Microsurgery, Kleinert Kutz
Hand Care Center, University of Louisville,
Louisville, Kentucky

ESTEBAN URRUTIA, MD
Clinical Fellow, Department of Orthopaedic
Surgery, School of Medicine, Pontificia
Universidad Católica de Chile, Santiago,
Chile

HARI VENKATRAMANI, MS, MCh (Plastic), DNB (Plastic), EDHS (Euro. Board)
Consultant Plastic Surgery, Department of Plastic, Hand & Reconstructive Microsurgery and Burns, Ganga Hospital, Coimbatore, Tamil Nadu, India

FU-CHAN WEI, MD, FACS
Distinguished Chair Professor, Department of Plastic and Reconstructive Surgery, Chang Gung Memorial Hospital, Chang Gung Medical College, Chang Gung University, Taipei, Taiwan

Contents

Mutilated injuries need to be treated aggressively and appropriately to avoid amputation or severe disability in the individual. Assessment of the management of these injuries on a global level reveals that there is a gap between the need and availability of the skilled manpower to manage these injuries. There is also a gap in the utilization of the available services. These gaps need to be covered or narrowed as far as possible. Although some measures need policy changes and improvement of health care delivery infrastructure, simpler measures taken at the final health care delivery level can significantly improve the final outcome.

Surgeons managing mutilating hand injures are faced with difficult decisions between attempting to salvage remaining or injured digits or proceeding to amputation and fusion. Through application of a basic understanding of hand biomechanics, the surgeon may more accurately predict what motion and function can best be salvaged. This article provides an explanation of how amputation, fusion, and tendon loss can affect postoperative hand motion. The surgeon can use these concepts in planning the reconstruction or preparing the foundation for secondary reconstructive procedures to achieve the highest functional outcome for the patient.

Understanding the global burden of trauma, particularly upper extremity trauma, is necessary in addressing the need for surgical services. Critical to that mission is to understand, and accurately measure, disability and related disability-adjusted life-years from massive upper extremity trauma. The impact of these injuries is magnified when considering that they frequently occur to young people in prime working years. This article discusses these social and medical system issues and reviews components of a comprehensive approach to measuring outcomes after these injuries. Patient-reported outcomes are highlighted. Methods of optimizing outcomes measurements and studies, disability assessments, and associated research are also discussed.

hand, the status of the remaining digits must be carefully assessed. Toe transfers, osteoplastic thumb reconstruction, and pollicization are commonly used. This article summarizes the indications and technical considerations in addressing the deficiencies after thumb amputation.

The metacarpal-like and metacarpal hand injuries are devastating conditions that render the hand nonfunctional. Although the metacarpal hand is well-studied, the metacarpal-like hand is never addressed. The authors, using the same principles as in the classification and treatment of metacarpal hand, propose an easy to follow treatment algorithm for metacarpal-like hand injury to guide the reconstructive surgeon. For both injuries, microsurgical toe-to-hand transplantation can restore an acceptable level of function if done properly. Meticulous planning is essential for the toe-to-hand surgery to achieve its prime goal of stable tripod pinch with insignificant morbidity at the donor sites.

Care of the reconstructed hand following mutilating injury is akin to the care of a vintage car. Its mechanisms are delicate, spare parts are limited, touch-ups are required often, and a major overhaul is indicated rarely. Secondary interventions are indicated for completion of staged primary procedures, management of complications, targeted improvement of function, and enhancement of appearance of the reconstructed hand. The approach to secondary reconstruction depends on the patient's age, and vocational and recreational requirements. It is also influenced by the constant evolution of surgeons' reconstructive philosophy, experience, and technology.

Management of mutilating hand injury is a challenge for any hand surgeon. Delay in presentation makes management even more challenging, usually because of inadequate initial assessment, inadequate debridement leading to infection, and secondary loss of tissues from exposure and desiccation. The aim is to obtain a functional hand by radical debridement, adequate assessment of the injury, appropriately timed reconstruction, and physiotherapy and rehabilitation. The hand surgeon must pay attention to the appearance of the hand by elimination of deformities, unsightly scars and bulky flaps to help to restore confidence in the patient to face the demands of daily living.

With the available microsurgical techniques, salvage of the limb can almost always provide a useful upper limb, even in the most complex combined injuries. Having a low threshold for revascularization of doubtfully viable extremities and making full use of the current armamentarium of soft tissue cover techniques, including flow through free flaps, will salvage many limbs. Secondary procedures, including free functioning muscle transfers and toe transfers, further increase the possible functional outcome. Even in the most complex combined injuries, intelligent reconstruction will obtain better outcomes than the best available prosthesis, making the efforts of salvage worthwhile.

HAND CLINICS

THE CLINICS ARE AVAILABLE ONLINE!
Access your subscription at:
www.theclinics.com

HAND CLINICS

Preface
Reconstructing Lives

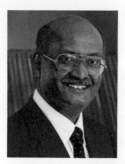

S. Raja Sabapathy, MS (Gen), MCh (Plastic),
DNB (Plastic), FRCS (Edin), MAMS
Editor

Reconstructing Lives—that is what we hand surgeons do when we work on a mutilated hand. Mutilating hand injuries are just not medical problems. It could mean loss of skills learned diligently over many years. In bilateral injuries, it could mean dependence on others for day-to-day activities and a loss of self-esteem. If it strikes a sole breadwinner of the family, in some parts of the world it could mean a social catastrophe. The management of these injuries demands the best of the skills of the hand surgeon. Any compromise in decision making or in execution of the procedure can significantly affect the ultimate functional outcome.

I thank the series editor Dr Kevin Chung for choosing the title of management of mutilated hand injuries, which is relevant to hand surgeons all over the world. In developing economies, unfortunately, this is a common injury. Appropriate care rendered in time is essential to get them back to work. Quality care is important to prevent complications. It is a health care burden that these countries can ill afford. In the western world, there is a low incidence of mutilating hand injuries, but they do occur. The mere lack of exposure to the demands of a mutilated hand will be a challenge to the surgeon who occasionally has to manage them. Pearls of wisdom of the experienced will serve as valuable sign posts. This issue contains material that will interest every hand surgeon.

It has been my privilege to be the editor of this issue. An opportunity was taken to get the views of renowned experts from across the world so that the pool of current knowledge will be made available to the hand surgery community. All the authors have put into words the lessons learned over the decades in managing mutilating hand injuries so that this issue will be a resource for anyone called to manage such injuries. An international perspective is provided. Working on these injuries for over three decades has convinced me that, in addition to the technical aspects of surgery, availability and accessibility of appropriate care play an important role in the management of mutilated hands. This issue of *Hand Clinics* starts by highlighting that factor, and the subsequent articles discuss the factors that are determinants of functional outcome.

It is the sincere hope of the editors and the contributors that the international perspective presented will serve as a resource for surgeons managing mutilated hands. If the contents presented in this issue help surgeons meet the challenges posed by these complex hand injuries and get a better functional outcome in these unfortunate patients, all our efforts will be worthwhile.

S. Raja Sabapathy, MS (Gen), MCh (Plastic)
DNB (Plastic), FRCS (Edin), MAMS
Division of Plastic Surgery, Hand Surgery
Reconstructive Microsurgery and Burns
Ganga Hospital
313, Mettupalayam Road
Coimbatore, Tamil Nadu
India 641 043

E-mail address:
rajahand@gmail.com

Hand Clin 32 (2016) xiii
http://dx.doi.org/10.1016/j.hcl.2016.08.011
0749-0712/16/© 2016 Published by Elsevier Inc.

hand.theclinics.com

Setting the Goals in the Management of Mutilated Injuries of the Hand—Impressions Based on the Ganga Hospital Experience

S. Raja Sabapathy, MS (Gen), MCh (Plastic), DNB (Plastic), FRCS (Edin), MAMS[a],*,
Praveen Bhardwaj, MS (Ortho), DNB (Ortho), FNB (Hand & Microsurgery), EDHS[b]

KEYWORDS

- Mutilated hand injuries management • Transfer of injured patients • Primary care of hand injuries
- Accessibility of quality health care • Cost of hand injury care

KEY POINTS

- Mutilated upper limb injuries if not treated appropriately end up in amputation or with severe disability to the individual.
- Making quality care available at the time of need is the key to success. It is desirable to set the following goals in the management of these injuries to achieve consistent good outcomes:
  - Goal 1: mutilated hand injuries must reach the appropriate center for their primary care.
  - Goal 2: experienced surgeons must be available at the time of primary decision making.
  - Goal 3: quality care must be made accessible to all patients with mutilated hand injuries irrespective of the socioeconomic status.
  - Goal 4: cost containment measures must be practiced to provide affordable services in the management of mutilated hand Injuries.

INTRODUCTION

Mutilated hand injury is a complex injury wherein there is injury to or loss of multiple tissue components in the upper limb. The bone is almost always fractured and there may be urgent need to vascularize the distal part. Unless treated effectively, there is a risk of amputation or for the individual to spend the rest of his life with severe disability. This possibility has not changed with time. So what has changed? First, there are more data on the outcome of efforts at salvage of these complex injuries to plan the strategy of management.[1–12]

Second, these injuries need high skill levels, and matching the availability of such skilled work force to the need in various parts of the world has become a challenge. Third, the cost of care has become an important issue in all health care systems and provision of cost-effective services has again become a challenge.[13–17]

With industrialization, work-related injuries contributed the greatest number of mutilated hand injuries. The enforcement of safety standards has thankfully reduced the injuries not only in the Western world but also in the developing world.[18]

[a] Division of Plastic Surgery, Hand Surgery, Reconstructive Microsurgery and Burns, Ganga Hospital, 313, Mettupalayam Road, Coimbatore, Tamil Nadu 641 043, India; [b] Hand & Wrist Surgery and Reconstructive Microsurgery, Ganga Hospital, 313, Mettupalayam Road, Coimbatore, Tamil Nadu 641 043, India
* Corresponding author.
E-mail address: rajahand@gmail.com

Hand Clin 32 (2016) 435–441
http://dx.doi.org/10.1016/j.hcl.2016.07.001
0749-0712/16/© 2016 Elsevier Inc. All rights reserved.

Even in India, work-related injuries are showing a diminishing trend. This positive development is offset by the increasing number of injuries that happen due to road traffic accidents. To this number needs to be added the severe injuries that happen in the operating room of war and terrorism. Because these injuries happen mostly to young people in the productive phases of their lives, effort to provide good care becomes worthwhile.

THE GOAL OF MANAGEMENT

The goal of management of a mutilated limb injury is to get a patient to preinjury status as early as possible. Because mutilated injuries often are associated with loss of tissue, reaching preinjury status may not be possible in many instances. The injuries are diverse and may pose a great challenge that a hand surgeon should be capable of handling.[19,20] Such injuries need all the skills of a hand surgeon, ranging from bone fixation to complex microsurgical flap cover and reconstruction. del Piñal[21,22] has suggested that an ideal scenario — the acceptable hand as one that has a thumb and at least three fingers of the correct length with motion at the proximal interphalangeal joint preserved along with sensation. This ideal, in many situations, may not be achievable. According to Moran and Berger[23] the minimal requirements for the hand are a stable wrist and 2 opposing sensate and painless digits. For digital requirements, only 1 digit requires motion, whereas the other can be a stable post, but both digits must be stable to withstand the force required to generate pinch. To accommodate larger objects and allow for prehensile movement, a cleft must be present between digits. Moran and Berger[23] also detail what is lost when the various components of the hand are lost. Having this idea guides salvaging components of the hand when possible and also aims at restoring function by secondary reconstruction.

Functional restoration has to be achieved at an affordable cost in the prevailing health care systems and patients have to be rehabilitated as early as possible.[24] Achieving these 2 objectives involves demands on infrastructure, availability of manpower, and logistics in administration.

The Health Care Paradigm

Effectiveness of health care delivery can be analyzed by the gaps that exist between health care need, availability, and utilization (Fig. 1). It is almost impossible to match these three in any disease management in most health care systems. The narrower the gap, the better the delivery of care. Bridging the gap between the need and

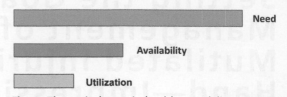

Fig. 1. The typical gaps in health care delivery status. Bridging gaps between need, availability, and utilization is the goal in the management of mutilated hand injuries.

availability requires efforts of high magnitude in infrastructure development and training and staffing of skilled workforce and may involve huge financial outlay, which needs the commitment of the government leadership and policy pronouncements and is a long-term target. Bridging the gap between availability and utilization is simpler and can be done by institution of protocols, set practices, and education. Much of it can be done by health care professionals and administrators and early measurable results can be achieved. Narrowing the gaps is again the goal in mutilated injury management.

A dedicated hand injury service was set up at Ganga Hospital in the Tier 2 city of Coimbatore, South India, in 1991 and gradually it has developed into a tertiary-level trauma care center. Approximately 6000 hand surgical procedures, including 51 replantations, 91 critical revascularizations, and 255 free tissue transfers, were done in the year 2015. The unit had a humble beginning and an analysis of the factors that made it successful has revealed that making some protocol changes could help in setting up a center of high volume wherein high-quality care can be delivered at an affordable cost—they are enumerated.

Goal 1: Mutilated Hand Injuries Must Reach the Appropriate Center for Their Primary Care

Experience in managing mutilated hand injury has taught that the ultimate outcome depends on the quality of initial débridement and primary skeletal stabilization, which lay the foundation for early soft tissue cover. If an injured limb requires revascularization, the needs become emergent. All these factors are dependent on the primary treating surgeon. When the injury happens, the decision, Where to go? becomes important because time is crucial in many instances (Fig. 2). After an amputation, the chances of replantation being attempted and the success rate depend on the center treating the patient. This finding is based on experience worldwide.[25–27] Shale and colleagues,[28] after a nationwide review, in the United

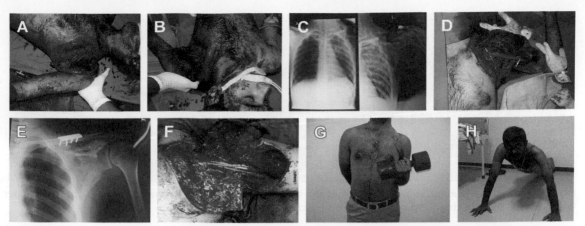

Fig. 2. (*A, B*) A patient who has suffered subtotal amputation of the left upper limb at the level of the shoulder. (*C*) Radiograph shows scapulo thoracic dissociation. The patient directly reached the center from the scene of the accident within 30 minutes of injury. (*D, E*) Skeletal stabilization achieved by the simple measure of clavicular plating. (*F*) The gap in the ruptured axillary artery was bridged by a vein graft. Limb revascularisation and the entire procedure was completed in 4 hours. (*G, H*) The patient subsequently had nerve transfers for shoulder abduction and elbow flexion to obtain a good functional outcome.

States, of the treatment patterns of traumatic thumb amputations, found that being in a teaching hospital increased the odds of attempted replantation by a factor of 3.1 (*P*<.001) compared with a nonteaching hospital. Treatment at a high-volume hospital increased the rate of attempted replantation by a factor of 3.3 (*P*<.001) compared with low-volume hospitals. Nylander and colleagues[29] in Finland found that replantation would have been technically possible in more than 70% of the cases, but attempts at replantation were only carried out in less than 10% of the serious cases. Worldwide, the experience is the same and has not changed over a long period of time.[30]

For obtaining better outcomes in mutilated hand injury management, the first goal is to raise the awareness among ambulance services and emergency rooms in the region of the availability of services and the need for early transfer to the appropriate center. Delay has meant disaster in many instances. If patients are fit for transport, the patients with mutilated hand injury have a chance of better outcome if they reach the appropriate center.[31] Scoop-and-run protocol rather than stay and play has worked in most instances.[32] Utilization of secure information technology solutions has helped surgeons who first see a patient to consult and decide on the transfer, and they have to be used liberally.[33]

When mutilated hand injuries occur as part of polytrauma, there is a possibility that the hand injury may not get the appropriate attention in the face of other life-threatening injuries.[34–36] Sometimes the mutilated hand injury does not get any treatment at all. If infection sets, in poor outcome is obtained. Life before limb is the right policy in polytrauma situations, but the limb injury must be attended to after the life-threatening injury is taken care of. Even in polytrauma situations, after the life-threatening injuries are attended to, debridement and skeletal fixation must be done on day 1 as far as possible. Established trauma systems have been shown of benefit in getting better outcomes after major trauma, due to the high volume and preparedness in treating such injuries. The same applies to mutilated injury management. Every center managing these injuries should take considerable effort at educating the ambulance service staff, emergency room personnel, and even the public on the need to reach the appropriate center early to get the best possible outcome. The goal is to make it happen in every instance.

Goal 2: Experienced Surgeons Must be Available at the Time of Primary Decision Making

Mutilated hand injury results in loss of various components. There are no predictable scoring systems to decide on salvage or amputation in upper limb injuries, so what matters are the experience and decision of the primary treating surgeon.[37–44] Experience allows a person to decide on salvage, possible heterotopic replantation, and utilization of valuable tissues as spare parts to get a better outcome (**Fig. 3**). In proximal injuries, decision making in salvage becomes more important because there are no good options for secondary reconstruction after amputation. Decision to salvage is also influenced by the possibility of obtaining a good

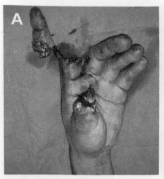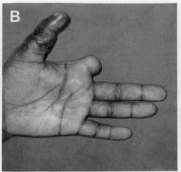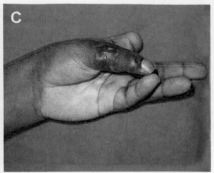

Fig. 3. (*A*) Total crush amputation of the thumb and the index finger. (*B, C*) The available part of the index finger is replanted over the thumb to make the hand functional.

functional outcome with the use of secondary procedures, like tendon transfers, selective arthrodesis, and free functional muscle transfers.[45] An experienced surgeon is able to visualize the end result and the pathway, which influence the primary surgery in many ways. Although good débridement forms the basis for reconstruction and most centers can do that, having the total plan influences the type of skeletal fixation, positioning of the external fixator pins, and the type and extent of flap cover. When later tendon transfers are needed, having the plan on hand during primary treatment helps design the flap cover so that it covers the entire pathway of the transfer. Often the authors have been struck by skin grafted patches between flaps that hamper the secondary procedure.

Primary or early referral to an appropriate center where senior surgeon input is available is encouraged. The authors have propagated the idea among the peripheral centers to ask the question, "Will all the demands of the patient be met by the skills of the treating team and the available infrastructure from the beginning to the end?" The authors have encouraged retaining and treating patients if the answer to the question is an emphatic "Yes." If not, the authors have requested the centers to have a low threshold for immediate or earliest possible referral. Often, this factor is ignored and patients are treated by a surgical team and, when they reach a stage when progress is no longer possible, they are referred to experienced teams. At this stage, the authors find that many bridges have already been burnt, and many good options of reconstruction have been lost either because of infection or poor planning in skeletal fixation or soft tissue cover. This is a situation that cannot be afforded in the management of mutilated injuries of the hand.

Goal 3: Quality Care Must be Made Accessible to All Patients with Mutilated Hand Injuries

Although universal quality care seems a lofty ideal and a distant dream, nevertheless it has to be aimed at. Mutilated hand injuries have a predilection to affect an economically poorer section of society worldwide. Karl and colleagues[46] found that phalangeal and metacarpal fractures varied by socioeconomic status, which decreased with increasing socioeconomic status. No other fracture varied by economic background of the patients. The situation must be the same in major hand injuries also. Even in the developed world, economic status influences the decision making and the treatment plan for a particular patient.[47]

Poor safety standards in industry and nonimplementation of safety rules on the roads are the main cause of accidents and they are more common in the developing world where more than 80% of the population lives. Analysis of the needs of primary management leads to confirming that in most instances, the surgeon factors are the strongest to influence outcome. Skill levels of the surgical team and the attitude of the treating surgeon are the main determinants during primary care. Availability of operating room time is always a pressing issue in most centers round the world. Unfortunately, hand trauma is considered at a less urgent platform compared with obstetric, abdominal, and neurotrauma emergencies. A skilled surgical team by performing faster could negotiate for more operating room time.

With reduced incidence of such injuries in many countries, exposure becomes limited to the younger generation of surgeons in the Western world. So when they are faced with the problem of a mutilated hand injury, chances are that optimum treatment might not be possible. On the other hand, in the developing world, the system is overwhelmed by the number of patients who need to be treated, which stresses the system and results in suboptimal care. In both situations, skill levels of the surgical team and their attitude could make the difference, by optimizing the use of the available operating room time. Skill comes with experience, so exposure of junior surgeons to high-volume hospitals for varying periods of time is crucial to build up the required experience. Although the surgeons of the developed world need numbers for training, the surgeons of the developing world need exposure to surgical techniques and instrumentation. Institution of fellowships and promotion of travel for teaching and training are key to progress in this field.

Goal 4: Cost Containment Procedures Must be Practiced in the Management of Mutilated Hand Injuries

Cost of care is an important issue in all health care systems. Mutilated hand injuries are expensive to treat, and poor treatment is more expensive because of the increased indirect cost in terms of number of days lost at work, loss of employment, and productivity. An internal audit at the authors' institution showed that 3 factors influence the cost of care. One is the incidence of complications, the most important being deep infection. Deep infection increases the cost of care by increasing hospital stay and days of antibiotic usage. Infection also delays secondary procedures and starting of rehabilitation. Most often deep infection is due to poor quality débridement. So radical débridement has to be stressed all the time and is the key to success in all reconstructive efforts. The second factor is performing primary reconstruction versus staged reconstruction. Coverage of critical raw areas by provision of flap cover on day 1, after débridement and skeletal fixation, reduced the overall cost of care by 25%, due to the reduced number of operating room visits and days of hospital stay. There was no increased incidence of infection in this protocol, which is possible if senior-level input is available on day 1. Provision of skin cover, even 48 to 72 hours later, does not affect infection rates but significantly affects the cost of care. The third factor is the institution of regional anesthesia practices over general anesthesia services. In the authors' center, 78% of hand trauma procedures were done under regional anesthesia techniques. Brachial blocks were combined with spinal or a combination of spinal and epidural anesthesia when flaps were raised from lower limb. Because mutilated hand injuries many times consume long operating hours, there is significant saving in terms of cost by exclusively using regional anesthesia practices. Consistent use of regional anesthesia has helped the authors push the boundaries, and even pediatric free flaps are done under regional anesthesia with comfort and huge reduction in cost of care.[48]

SUMMARY

Numerous studies with long-term follow-up have proved the advantage of salvage of amputated limbs by replantation over amputation. Although this is the case with replantation, subtotal amputations and reconstructed mutilated limbs where some tissues are in continuity must fare much better. There does not seem to be any alternative for good reconstruction in the present state for upper limb injuries. Prosthesis technology is yet to catch up with the outcome achieved by a well-reconstructed upper limb.[49,50] Now there are long-term results to compare replants with hand transplantation. Because transplantation scores positive points in bilateral amputations, and most mutilated hands are unilateral, automatically salvage options become more important.[51,52]

The goal must be to provide patients the best care offered today, which is reached by practicing a series of steps in the right sequence and paying attention to detail. In addition, every effort must be taken to make the expertise available to every patient who needs it and at the time it is needed.

REFERENCES

1. O'Reilly GM, Gabbe B, Moore L, et al. Classifying, measuring and improving the quality of data in trauma registries: A review of the literature. Injury 2016;47(3):559–67.
2. Dias JJ, Chung KC, Garcia-Elias M, et al. Recommendations for the improvement of hand injury care across the world. Injury 2006;37(11):1078–82.
3. Chan J, Spencer J. Adaptation to hand injury: an evolving experience. Am J Occup Ther 2004;58(2):128–39.
4. Stanger K, Horch RE, Dragu A. Severe mutilating injuries with complex macroamputations of the upper extremity - is it worth the effort? World J Emerg Surg 2015;7(10):30.
5. Hudak PL, Amadio PC, Bombardier C. Development of an upper extremity outcome measure: the DASH (disabilities of the arm, shoulder and hand) [corrected]. The Upper Extremity Collaborative Group (UECG). Am J Ind Med 1996;29(6):602–8.

6. Guyatt GH, Feeny DH, Patrick DL. Measuring health-related quality of life. Ann Intern Med 1993;118(8): 622–9.

7. Barbier O, Penta M, Thonnard JL. Outcome evaluation of the hand and wrist according to the International Classification of Functioning, Disability, and Health. Hand Clin 2003;19(3):371–8.

8. Gill TM, Feinstein AR. A critical appraisal of the quality of quality-of-life measurements. JAMA 1994; 272(8):619–26.

9. Sabapathy SR, Satbhai NG. Microsurgery in the urgent and emergent management of the hand. Curr Rev Musculoskelet Med 2014;7(1):40–6.

10. Fox-Rushby JA, Hanson K. Calculating and presenting disability adjusted life years (DALYs) in cost-effectiveness analysis. Health Policy Plan 2001; 16(3):326–31.

11. Alderman AK, Chung KC. Measuring outcomes in hand surgery. Clin Plast Surg 2008;35(2):239–50.

12. Chung KC, Hamill JB, Walters MR, et al. The Michigan Hand Outcomes Questionnaire (MHQ): assessment of responsiveness to clinical change. Ann Plast Surg 1999;42(6):619–22.

13. Dias JJ, Garcia-Elias M. Hand injury costs. Injury 2006;37(11):1071–7.

14. Holmberg J, Lindgren B, Jutemark R. Replantation-revascularization and primary amputation in major hand injuries. Resources spent on treatment and the indirect costs of sick leave in Sweden. J Hand Surg 1996;21(5):576–80.

15. de Putter CE, Selles RW, Polinder S, et al. Economic impact of hand and wrist injuries: health-care costs and productivity costs in a population-based study. J Bone Joint Surg Am 2012;94(9):e56.

16. Omoke NI, Chukwu CO, Madubueze CC, et al. Traumatic extremity amputation in a Nigerian setting: patterns and challenges of care. Int Orthop 2012; 36(3):613–8.

17. Trybus M, Lorkowski J, Brongel L, et al. Causes and consequences of hand injuries. Am J Surg 2006; 192(1):52–7.

18. Ernstberger A, Joeris A, Daigl M, et al. Decrease of morbidity in road traffic accidents in a high income country - an analysis of 24,405 accidents in a 21 year period. Injury 2015;46(Suppl 4):S135–43.

19. Burkhalter W. Mutilating injuries of the hand. Hand Clin 1986;2:45–68.

20. Midgley RD, Entin MA. Management of mutilating injuries of the hand. Clin Plast Surg 1976;3(1):99–109.

21. del Piñal F. Severe mutilating injuries to the hand: guidelines for organizing the chaos. J Plast Reconstr Aesthet Surg 2007;60(7):816–27.

22. del Piñal F. The indications for toe transfer after "minor" finger injuries. J Hand Surg Br 2004;29(2): 120–9.

23. Moran SL, Berger RA. Biomechanics and hand trauma: what you need. Hand Clin 2003;19:17–31.

24. Sabapathy SR, Bhardwaj P. Microsurgery and complex hand injuries. In: Cheema TA, editor. Complex injuries of the hand. London: JP Medical Publishers; 2014. p. 233–54.

25. Friedrich JB, Poppler LH, Mack CD, et al. Epidemiology of upper extremity replantation surgery in the United States. J Hand Surg Am 2011; 36(11):1835–40.

26. Chang DH, Ye SY, Chien LC, et al. Epidemiology of Digital Amputation and Replantation in Taiwan - A Population-Based Study. Plast Reconstr Surg 2015; 136(4 Suppl):27–8.

27. Sabapathy SR, Venkatramani H. Massive upper limb trauma. In: Trail IA, Fleming ANM, editors. Disorder of the hand. London: Springer; 2015. p. 391–414.

28. Shale CM, Tidwell JE 3rd, Mulligan RP, et al. A nationwide review of the treatment patterns of traumatic thumb amputations. Ann Plast Surg 2013;70(6):647–51.

29. Nylander G, Vilkki S, Ostrup L. The need for replantation surgery after traumatic amputations of the upper extremity–an estimate based upon the epidemiology of Sweden. J Hand Surg Br 1984; 9(3):257–60.

30. Sabapathy R. Management of complex injuries and replantation across the world. Injury 2006;37(11): 1057–60.

31. Nirula R, Maier R, Moore E, et al. Scoop and run to the trauma center or stay and play at the local hospital: hospital transfer's effect on mortality. J Trauma 2010;69(3):595–9.

32. Smith RM, Conn AK. Prehospital care - scoop and run or stay and play? Injury 2009;40(Suppl 4):S23–6.

33. Hustedt JW, Bohl DD, Champagne L. The Detrimental Effect of Decentralization in Digital Replantation in the United States: 15 Years of Evidence From the National Inpatient Sample. J Hand Surg Am 2016;41(5):593–601.

34. Blum J, Gercek E, Hansen M, et al. Operative strategies in the treatment of upper limb fractures in poly-traumatized patients. Unfallchirurgie 2005;108(10): 843–9 [in German].

35. Enweluzo GO, Giwa SO, Obalum DC. Pattern of extremity injuries in polytrauma in Lagos, Nigeria. Niger Postgrad Med J 2008;15(1):6–9.

36. Rubin G, Peleg K, Givon A, Israel Trauma Group. Upper extremity fractures among hospitalized pediatric road traffic accident victims. Am J Emerg Med 2015;33(5):667–70.

37. Hentz VR, Chase RA. The Philosophy of Hand Salvage and Repair. In: Wolfort FG, editor. Acute Hand Inuries - a multispecialty approach. Boston (MA): Little, Brown; 1980. p. 1–26.

38. Lin CH, Webb K, Neumeister MW. Immediate tissue transplantation in upper limb trauma: spare parts reconstruction. Clinplast Surg 2014;41(3): 397–406.

39. Togawa S, Yamami N, Nakayama H, et al. The validity of the mangled extremity severity score in the assessment of upper limb injuries. J Bone Joint Surg Br 2005;87(11):1516–9.

40. Prichayudh S, Verananvattna A, Sriussadaporn S, et al. Management of upper extremity vascular injury: outcome related to the Mangled Extremity Severity Score. World J Surg 2009; 33(4):857–63.

41. Brown HC, William HB, Woodhouse FM. Principles of salvage in mutilating hand injuries. J Trauma 1968;8: 319–32.

42. McCormack RM. Reconstructive surgery and the immediate care of the severely injured hand. Clin Orthop 1959;13:75–82.

43. Graham B, Adkins P, Tsai TM, et al. Major replantation versus revision amputation and prosthetic fitting in the upper extremity: a late functional outcomes study. J Hand Surg Am 1998;23(5): 783–91.

44. Peacock K, Tsai TM. Comparison of functional results of replantation versus prosthesis in a patient with bilateral arm amputation. Clin Orthop Relat Res 1987;214:153–9.

45. Sabapathy SR, Bhardwaj P. Secondary procedures in replantation. Semin Plast Surg 2013; 27(4):198–204.

46. Karl JW, Olson PR, Rosenwasser MP. The Epidemiology of Upper Extremity Fractures in the United States, 2009. J Orthop Trauma 2015;29(8):e242–4.

47. Mahmoudi E, Squitieri L, Maroukis BL, et al. Care transfers for patients with upper extremity trauma: influence of health insurance type. J Hand Surg Am 2016;41(4):516–25.

48. Bjorklund KA, Venkatramani H, Venkateshwaran G, et al. Regional anesthesia alone for pediatric free flaps. J Plast Reconstr Aesthet Surg 2015;68(5): 705–8.

49. Schneeberger S, Gorantla VS, Hautz T, et al. Immunosuppression and rejection in human hand transplantation. Transplant Proc 2009;41(2): 472–5.

50. Gorantla VS, Demetris AJ. Acute and chronic rejection in upper extremity transplantation: what have we learned? Hand Clin 2011;27(4):481–93.

51. Breidenbach WC, Meister EA, Turker T, et al. A Methodology for Determining Standard of Care Status for a New Surgical Procedure: Hand Transplantation. Plast Reconstr Surg 2016;137(1):367–73.

52. Breidenbach WC, Meister EA, Hassan K. Discussion: perceptions of the risks and benefits of upper limb transplantation among individuals with upper limb amputations. Plast Reconstr Surg 2014; 134(5):988–9.

The Biomechanical Impact of Digital Loss and Fusion Following Trauma
Setting the Patient up for Success

Heather L. Baltzer, MSc, MD, FRCS(C)[a],
Steven L. Moran, MD[b,c],*

KEYWORDS

- Digital amputation • Digital replantation • Mutilating hand trauma • Hand biomechanics

KEY POINTS

- An understanding of normal hand biomechanics and the implications of digital loss or fusion are important for intraoperative decision making after mutilating hand injury.
- Minimal requirements for the hand are a stable wrist and 2 opposing sensate digits.
- In this article, we outline 7 basic hand functions; however, the preservation of thumb-finger pinch and digito-palmar grip have priority.
- Patients with mutilating hand injuries often require secondary procedures and these should be considered at the initial reconstructive attempt so as to set the stage appropriately.
- Future directions pertain to understanding the implications of fusion, the role of arthroplasty, free-toe transfer, prosthetics, and hand transplantation following these devastating injuries.

INTRODUCTION

Mutilating hand injuries continue to present challenges for the hand surgeon and patient. The surgeon must often make decisions at the time of initial debridement with regards to finger and joint preservation and the appropriate use of spare parts. A solid understanding of the biomechanical sequelae of amputation and fusion is critical for making appropriate decisions in these circumstances. In 2003, we published an article highlighting the biomechanical impact of immediate amputation and fusion following hand trauma.[1] In this update, we evaluate many of these issues

with a focus on new developments and advances in joint replacement, microsurgery, and hand transplantation as they relate to mutilating hand trauma.

Mutilating hand injuries vary in extent and severity. To guide the hand surgeon in generating an organized approach to these injuries, several grading scales, and algorithms have been developed.[2–7] Although algorithms can assist in surgical planning, no grading scale has been consistently correlated with postreconstructive hand function. Heroic attempts are made to save digits that become stiff and painful postoperatively, impeding hand function. In retrospect, the loss of a single

Disclosure Statement: Dr H.L. Baltzer has no disclosures. Dr S.L. Moran is a paid consultant for Integra Life Sciences.
a Toronto Western Hand Program, University Health Network, University of Toronto, 399 Bathurst Street, 2nd Floor East Wing, Room 422, Toronto, Ontario M5T 2S8, Canada; b Division of Orthopedic Surgery, Department of Hand Surgery, Mayo Clinic, 200 1st Street Southwest, Rochester, MN 55905, USA; c Division of Plastic Surgery, Mayo Clinic, 200 1st Street Southwest, Rochester, MN 55905, USA
* Corresponding author. Division of Plastic Surgery, Mayo Clinic, 200 1st Street Southwest, Rochester, MN 55905.
E-mail address: moran.steven@mayo.edu

Hand Clin 32 (2016) 443–463
http://dx.doi.org/10.1016/j.hcl.2016.07.003
0749-0712/16/© 2016 Elsevier Inc. All rights reserved.

digit or joint may not result in a significant functional deficit. Despite this fact, intraoperative decision making can still be agonizing for the hand surgeon to anticipate precisely the functional implications of immediate joint fusion or amputation, particularly for the young hand surgeon with limited experience. To begin to consider what needs to be saved it is best to begin thinking about the basic elements of hand function.

THE ESSENTIALS

Minimal requirements for the hand are a stable wrist and 2 opposing sensate digits. If the wrist is unstable, all flexion and extension forces generated by the forearm muscles will be dissipated across the wrist, making finger motion ineffective. For digital requirements, only 1 digit requires motion, whereas the other can be a stable post, but both digits must be stable to withstand the force required to generate pinch. To accommodate larger objects and allow for prehensile movement, a cleft must be present between digits. Above all else, sensate and pain-free digits are necessary for a reconstructed hand to be functional; otherwise, they provide little benefit over prosthesis.[8-10] A 2-point discrimination of less than 10 to 12 mm has been defined as functional sensation (**Figs. 1** and **2**).[11]

Prehension, as defined by Tubiana and Mackin,[12] is "as all the functions that are put into play when an object is grasped by the hands—intent, permanent sensory control, and a mechanism of grip." Prehension simply means the ability to grasp and manipulate objects. There are 3 components of prehension: the ability to approach, grasp, and release an object.[12,13] These 3 functions can be accomplished

(and enable prehension) even if only 2 sensate digits remain to oppose each other (see **Figs. 1** and **2**).

The hand's functions can be broken down to 7 basic maneuvers, which have been previously described.[1] These include the following:

1. Precision pinch (terminal pinch). This involves flexion at the distal interphalangeal (DIP) joint of the index and at the interphalangeal joint (IP) joint of the thumb. The ends of the fingernails are brought together as in lifting a paper clip from a tabletop (**Fig. 3**A).
2. Key pinch. The thumb is adducted to the radial side of the middle phalanx of the index finger. Requirements for key pinch include a stable post (usually the index finger of adequate length) and a stable thumb metacarpal phalangeal (MP) joint, which can resist the force of adductor pollicis (**Fig. 3**B).
3. Oppositional pinch (subterminal pinch). The pulp of the index and thumb are brought together with the DIP joints extended. Requirements for oppositional pinch force to be generated include thumb opposition, first dorsal interosseous contraction, and index profundus flexion. This motion can be measured using a dynamometer (**Fig. 3**C).
4. Directional grip (chuck grip). The thumb, index, and long finger come together to surround a cylindrical object to generate a rotational and axial force applied to the held object (ie, using a screwdriver) (**Fig. 3**D). This usually requires the presence of a thumb, 2 fingers, and a functional distal radio-ulnar joint.
5. Hook grip. The combination of MP joint extension and IP joint flexion of the fingers to transmit a unidirectional force (eg, pulling a door handle)

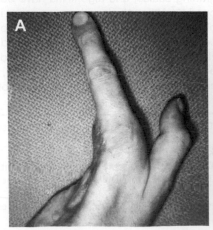
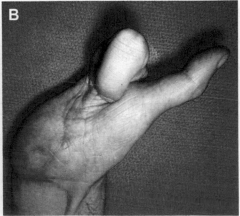

Fig. 1. The rudimentary hand contains a stable wrist and 2 opposable digits. The digits should be pain-free and sensate.

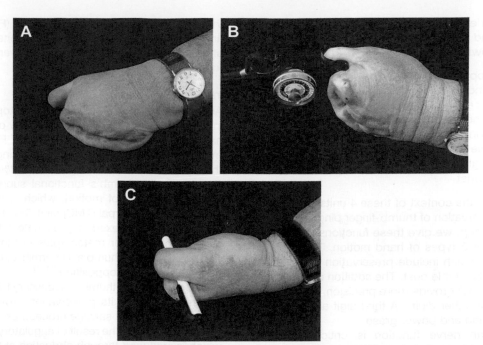

Fig. 2. Despite the loss of most of the digits, this hand remains functional for this patient because it has a stable post (the remaining index finger), a web space, and a mobile thumb capable of generating pinch force through adduction. This patient refused further surgery.

or to lift an object such as a suitcase. It is the only type of functional grasp that does not require thumb function (**Fig. 3**E).

6. Power grasp. The fingers are fully flexed at IP and MP joints while the thumb is flexed and opposed over the other digits, as in holding a hammer. Force is applied through the fingers into the palm (**Fig. 3**F).

7. Span grasp. The DIP and proximal interphalangeal (PIP) joints flex to approximately 30°, the MP joints are extended and fingers are abducted. The thumb is abducted. Force is generated between the thumb and fingers. Stability is required at the thumb MP and IP. This grip is used to lift cylindrical objects (**Fig. 3**G).[12,14,15]

The goal of the reconstructive procedure after a mutilating hand injury is to restore the hand's ability to adopt these positions and exert force through them. This recovery will be dependent on numerous factors, including the severity of the injury, the reconstruction, and the patient's compliance with rehabilitation postoperatively. In addition, it is critical to have restoration of functional sensation, particularly in the radial 3 digits for pinch.[3] Reconstructive goals should be based on the preoperative history and a knowledge of which hand functions will benefit the patient the most in returning to their previous employment or activities.

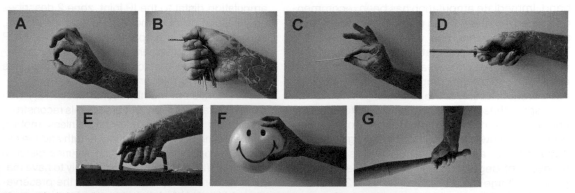

Fig. 3. The 7 basic hand functions. (*A*) Precision pinch (terminal pinch). (*B*) Key pinch. (*C*) Oppositional pinch (subterminal pinch). (*D*) Directional grip (chuck grip). (*E*) Hook grip. (*F*) Power grasp. (*G*) Span grasp.

When evaluating the mutilated hand, we break the hand into 4 functional units. These include the following:

1. The opposable thumb
2. The index and long finger, whose stable carpometacarpal (CMC) joints serve as fixed posts for pinch and power functions
3. The ring and small finger, which represent the mobile unit of the hand, with motion provided through their CMC joints
4. The wrist

Within the context of these 4 units we focus on the preservation of thumb-finger pinch and digito-palmar grip; we give these functions priority over the other 5 types of hand motion. The prerequisites for pinch include preservation of the thumb unit and a stable post. The addition of a third digit to pinch will provide more precision, as it can stabilize the other digit.[3] A third digit also allows for chuck grip and power grasp.

Median nerve function is critical for pinch involving the radial digits. Without median nerve function, both thumb sensation and most thenar muscle function is lost, making fine motor movements negligible. In contrast to pinch, digitopalmar grip requires preservation of ulnar nerve function and the ring-small finger unit to provide flexion and sensation in the ulnar digits. Interosseous function is necessary for stabilization of metacarpalphalangeal joint (MCP) motion and prevents clawing during object grasp and accommodation. Thumb preservation is also important in power grasp to provide stability and control of directional forces. These are the principles on which this article examines the implications of digital amputation and fusion on hand function.

The Biomechanical Impact of Amputation

Mutilating hand injuries nearly always result in partial or complete amputations at some level in the hand. Immediate amputation has been recommended when 4 of the 6 basic digital parts (bone, joint, skin, tendon, nerve, and vessel) are injured.[16–22] The rationale for immediate amputation is to prevent long-term stiffness and pain in a salvaged digit. Badly damaged fingers also may delay or impair rehabilitation of the remaining hand.

Despite these guidelines for amputation, it is important to remember that advances in microsurgery now allow for replantation of digits injured beyond the IP and DIP level, as well as functional recovery of degloved digits.[23–27] It is always our goal to salvage the thumb and at least 2 other fingers if possible. To preserve thumb function, ectopic replantation can be used to reconstruct a thumb from the best preserved digits (**Fig. 4**). If amputation needs to be performed, one should understand how digital loss affects overall hand function.[1,3]

Thumb amputation

Above all other digits, the thumb takes top priority in salvage.[28] The thumb provides 40% of overall hand function in the uninjured hand.[29–31] Following mutilating trauma, when digits are missing or stiff, the thumb can account for more than 50% of hand function.[32] The thumb's functional superiority is related to its axis of motion, which is based at the trapeziometacarpal (TMC) joint. The TMC joint is pronated and flexed approximately 80° with respect to the other metacarpals in the hand.[33] The position of the thumb axis permits circumduction, which permits opposition.[34–37]

Opposition of the thumb is necessary for all useful prehension and its preservation provides the basis for successful salvage procedures. Opposition of the thumb is the result of angulatory motion, which is produced through abduction at the TMC joint, and flexion and rotation of the TMC and MP joints.[38] Multiple muscles are required for functional opposition. These include the abductor pollicis brevis, the opponenspollicis, and the superficial head of the flexor pollicis brevis. These muscles act simultaneously on the TMC joint and the MP joint. The primary motor for thumb opposition is abductor pollicis brevis, with the opponens pollicis and flexor pollicis brevis providing secondary motors for opposition. The extensor pollicis longus (EPL) and adductor pollicis are antagonists to thumb opposition, providing a supinating extension and adduction force. Effort should be directed toward preserving or reconstructing the abductor pollicis brevis when possible, as this has the greatest cross-sectional area representing the strongest of the thenar muscles.[33,36–40]

Thumb amputation has been previously categorized into 5 zones[1] (**Fig. 5**). Briefly, zone 1 involves amputation distal to the IP joint, zone 2 describes amputations distal to the MCP joint to the IP joint, zone 3 describes amputations about the MCP joint, zone 4 injuries are extra-articular amputations through the metacarpal, and zone 5 injuries involve the TMC joint or proximal.

The priorities of thumb reconstruction vary with the level of amputation, but at all levels reconstruction should attempt to restore a painless, mobile, stable thumb that has adequate length and the capacity for opposition and pinch. Injuries distal to the IP joint (zone 1 injuries) are unlikely to have major limitations on opposition due to the preservation of length.[41,42] Injuries at this level are more likely to produce insensibility and dysesthesia

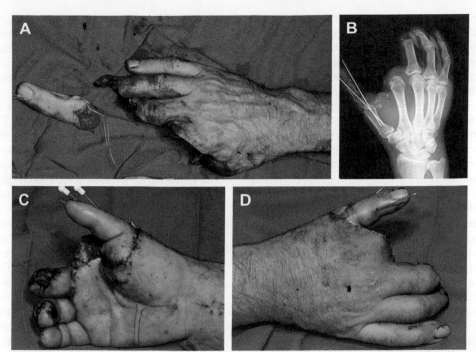

Fig. 4. Example of distal or ectopic replant in a 63-year-old man injured at work with a chop saw (*A*). The amputated thumb and long finger were too damaged for replantation so the remaining index finger was replanted onto the thumb stump in zone 3. The intact sesamoid bone, seen in the anteroposterior (AP) radiograph (*B*) of the native thumb, shows that the thenar muscles are intact. Image at 2 weeks with Kirschner wires still in place (*C, D*).

due to the trauma,[43,44] and can negatively impact subterminal pinch and precision pinch. Pinch can be compromised if an unstable or painful scar is present at the thumb remnant. Loss of the distal phalanx and IP joint (zone 2 injuries) may also not

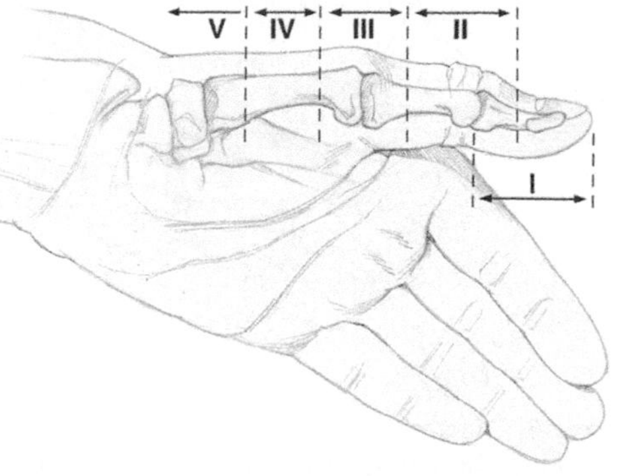

Fig. 5. Diagram depicting levels of thumb amputation. Zone I injuries involve the distal phalanx but spare the IP joint, zone II injuries involve the IP joint, zone III injuries involve the MP joint but spare the thenar muscles, zone IV injuries occur through the thumb metacarpal shaft, and zone V injuries involve damage or loss of the TMC joint. (*Courtesy of* Mayo Clinic; with permission.)

require reconstruction. Function may be preserved if both TMC and MP motion are maintained.[45]

The most common injuries are through the level of the MP joint (zone3), and will result in a significant loss of function. Unreconstructed injuries result in a decrease in pinch dexterity and grip strength.[46] The MP joint of the thumb has unique biomechanical properties in that it acts as a ball-and-socket joint in extension, but in flexion, the tight collateral ligaments act to allow the MP joint to function as a hinge. These properties produce 3° of freedom. The intrinsic muscles provide motion but also provide dynamic stability to the joint.

Injuries through the thumb MP joint are an indication for a free-toe transfer, which is the gold standard for amputations at this level. Compared with patients who do not have a thumb reconstruction, toe transfer can improve objective and subjective hand function scores.[47] When the injury is proximal to the MP joint, the great toe metatarsal phalangeal joint can reproduce the flexion and extension arc of the MP joint, but the toe MP joint fails to reproduce the thumb MP joints 15 to 20° of supination.[44] Other microsurgical options for reconstruction at this level include the toe wrap-around flap. This reconstruction only allows for TMC motion, but excellent results have been obtained from toe wrap-around reconstruction when the fusion angles with bone graft were 30° of flexion and 45° of internal rotation. These fusion angles have been shown to allow for pinch between all fingers and the reconstructed thumb. Additionally,[47] pinch and grip strengths can measure 60% and 97% of the contralateral side respectively.[48] A recent review of 3-year follow-up among patients who received toe transfer demonstrates that most patients can perform fine motor tasks without difficulty; pinch strength can be restored up to 75% of the contralateral hand[49] and grip strength can be restored to approximately 70% of the contralateral hand when performing an immediate second toe transfer, and up to 90% with wrap-around techniques.[26] Nonmicrosurgical methods for reconstruction of distal metacarpal thumb amputations can include metacarpal lengthening[50] and/or deepening of the first web space. The latter can produce injury to the adductor or thenar musculature, and as such, should be discouraged in an already traumatized thumb.

Level 4 injuries are at the level of the midshaft of the thumb metacarpal and result in damage to the thenar muscles. The sequela of this type of injury is loss of thenar function even if a free-toe transfer is performed. Toe transfers for this level of injury are usually accompanied by an opponensplasty to restore thumb opposition.[46,50,51] In its most primitive form, appositional pinch can be recreated, as in the tetraplegic patient, with fusion of the IP and MP joints and reconstruction of the adductor musculature; however, for reconstruction of oppositional pinch, tendon transfers are generally required.

For those requiring tendon transfers in the setting of trauma, the 2 main considerations for the surgeon are the choice of donor muscle and pulley location. The cross-sectional area and moment arm of flexor digitorum superficialis (FDS) of the long finger and the extensor carpi ulnaris (ECU) have been shown to have the closest approximation of thenar muscle strength and excursion.[35] Pulley location for oppositional transfers has been shown to influence the motion and strength of transfers in both the flexion and abduction planes. Both Bunnell[52] and Cooney and colleagues[35] stress the importance of directing the force of the transfer toward the pisiform. Oppositional transfers with a pulley located distal to the pisiform, such as the extensor digiti minimi (EDQ) or abductor digiti minimi transfer (ADQ), produce more flexion than abduction. Transfers with pulleys proximal to the pisiform, such as the FDS using the flexor carpi ulnaris (FCU) loop as a pulley, produce more palmar abduction and less metacarpal flexion. Other factors such as scaring and rehabilitation will certainly impact the results of opponensplasty success. A recent biomechanical study examining frictional

forces created during opponensplasty, demonstrated that a superficialis tendon transfer passed through Guyon's canal had the lowest friction and created the greatest opposition when compared with a palmar fascia pulley (Royal Thompson pulley) and FCU-based pullies.[53]

Zone 5 injuries represent a loss of, or injury to, the TMC joint. Historically, injury of the TMC joint has been an indication for index finger pollicization, due to the difficulties associated with TMC reconstruction. The TMC joint is mechanically equivalent to a universal joint allowing for thumb circumduction and extension with associated supination, and pronation with thumb flexion.[36,38,54] The TMC joint has inherent instability at the radial aspect of the wrist secondary to the lack of bony stabilizers proximally (mobile scaphoid) and the large cantilever forces exerted on it by the thumb. To counter this instability there is a complex network of over a dozen ligamentous supports that surround the joint, with 5 major internal ligamentous stabilizers: (1) dorsal radial ligament, (2) posterior oblique ligament, (3) first intermetacarpal ligament, (4) ulnar collateral ligament, and (5) the anterior oblique ligament (**Fig. 6**). The dorsal radial ligament prevents lateral subluxation. The posterior oblique ligament

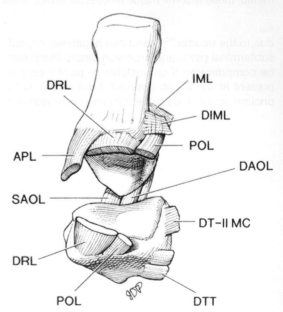

Fig. 6. Diagram of the trapezio-metacarpal joint showing the outlay of the dorsal and volar ligaments. Special attention must be given to preservation of this joint for adequate thumb stability. The most important ligaments for reconstruction and preservation are the dorsal radial ligament (DRL), posterior oblique ligament (POL), ulnar collateral ligament (not depicted), first intermetacarpal ligament (IML), and the anterior oblique ligament, deep and superficial heads (DAOL, SAOL, respectively). (*Courtesy of* Mayo Clinic; with permission.)

provides stability in flexion, opposition, and pronation. The first intermetacarpal ligament tethers the first metacarpal base to the second and becomes taut in abduction, opposition, and supination. The intermetacarpal ligament is joined by the ulnar collateral ligament, which prevents lateral subluxation of the first metacarpal on the trapezium and controls for rotational stress. As such, it is critical that the base of the index metacarpal is spared during any type of index ray resection to preserve the intermetacarpal ligament helping to stabilize the thumb.[55,56] It is believed that the most important ligament for thumb stabilization is the volar anterior oblique ligament that arises from the volar tubercle of the trapezium and inserts on the volar aspect of the metacarpal base. The superficial component of the anterior oblique ligament is taut in extension, abduction, and pronation; it controls pronation stress and prevents radial translation. The deep anterior oblique ligament serves as a pivot point for the TMC joint and guides the metacarpal into pronation while the thenar muscles work in concert to produce abduction and flexion. These fibers limit ulnar translocation of the metacarpal during palmer abduction while working with the superficial anterior oblique ligament to constrain volar subluxation of the metacarpal. The anterior oblique, intermetacarpal, and dorsoradial ligaments are the most critical for preservation and reconstruction.[54–56] Although reports of CMC reconstruction are limited, more recent results of free-toe reconstruction suggests that toe transfer for zone 5 injuries is possible, but little comparison data are available relative to index pollicization.[57–59] One study found limited indications for pollicization, mainly that function was relatively equivocal in thumb-only injuries, whereas it provided weak pinch in more complex hand juries.[60]

In summary: amputations of the thumb

In summary, the goals of thumb restoration are to maintain a painless, stable yet mobile thumb, with adequate length and the capacity for opposition. For zone 1 and 2 injuries, the goals of reconstruction should be to ensure a pain-free stump that is stable at the IP and MP joints respectively. Zone 3 injuries require restoration of length and mobility at the MP joint, best performed with a free-toe transfer. Zone 4 injuries will require restoration of length, with free-toe transfer and some form of tendon transfer for opposition, and zone 5 injuries will require all of the previously mentioned along with TMC mobility or some attempt at TMC reconstruction.

Index Finger Amputation

Although the order of priority of digit salvage is debated, the index finger may be of next-highest importance because of its flexion and extension independence, its ability to abduct, and its proximity to the thumb. It has a major role in precision pinch and directional grip.[12,14,61,62] The goal in index finger salvage is to maintain a good range of motion over preservation of length. A high level of success with good functional outcomes has been demonstrated after finger salvage for mangling index finger injures.[63] An amputation at the PIP level still allows for flexion of the remaining index stump to approximately 45° due to the remaining intrinsic function. Even if shortened to the distal end of the proximal phalanx, the index can still participate in directional grip, span grasp, and lateral pinch.[14] The brain, however, is quick to bypass the digit for the long finger if it becomes painful, insensate or stiff, which can make the index a hindrance to hand function.[64] The long finger replaces the index for terminal and subterminal pinch if index amputation is performed below the DIP level.

Elective loss of the index ray results in diminished power grip, key pinch, and supination strength by approximately 20% following surgery.[65] This loss of grip strength is accentuated in patients with persistent dysesthesia following ray amputation. In addition, pronation strength, important in directional grip, is diminished by 50% following ray resection. This large decrease in pronation strength is caused by a shortening of the palm's lever arm. In the intact hand, the width of the grip extends from the hypothenar region to the index finger. The ulnar aspect of the palm represents the internal fulcrum, and the radial aspect of the palm represents the external fulcrum of movement. The loss of the index finger ray decreases the fulcrum by approximately 25% (**Fig. 7**), resulting in a loss of stability and diminished mechanical advantage. Just as concerning as loss of strength, is the high prevalence of neuroma formation within the remaining first web space. Murray and colleagues[65] found that the most disabling complication following index ray resection was hyperesthesia, or painful sensitivity to light touch, in the thumb-long-finger web. This was present in 59% of patients and interfered with hand function in 37%. Interestingly, the minority of patients who healed without postoperative dysesthesia felt that their overall hand function had been improved with the removal of the index

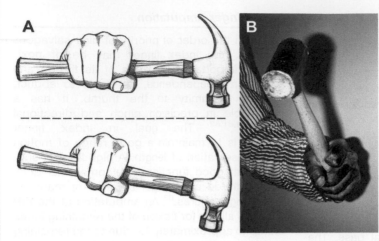

Fig. 7. Loss to the index finger with the index ray and MCP joint results in a 25% decrease in hand width; this in turn leads to a shortened lever arm decreasing pronation and supination strength (*A*). (*B*) Shows benefit of even a small portion of the index in stabilizing larger objects and preserving palm length. Flexion of the remaining index finger stump is provided by intact intrinsic function. (*Courtesy of* [*A*] Mayo Clinic; with permission.)

finger. This was related specifically to improved prehension between the thumb and long finger. These findings would suggest that prehensile function may be more important than preserved grip strength for certain patients. Other investigators believe that with second ray amputation, mobility of remaining rays improves through the CMC joints increasing function of the remaining digits.[64] A comparative study of patients with traumatic index amputations at the proximal phalanx level and patients with elective index ray resections demonstrated that patients receiving index amputation at the proximal phalanx level had better self-reported function based on DASH (Disabilities of the Arm, Shoulder, and Hand) scores. Cosmesis was believed to be better with ray amputation.[66] Although both groups demonstrated a 30% decrease in pinch and grip strength, it seems that a remaining proximal phalanx stump does provide a benefit in terms of grip strength and overall hand function. In light of the high rate of postoperative dysesthesia that can be associated with ray resection, it seems that immediate index ray resection should be reserved for very proximal injuries where there is little chance of postoperative MP motion or where soft tissue coverage is needed to preserve an adequate first web space. Recent studies have shown that patients with salvaged index fingers are 2 times more likely to have an unplanned operation in comparison with those who undergo immediate amputation. The authors stress the importance of shared decision making in these situations, as 1 in 5 repaired index fingers were eventually amputated (**Fig. 8**).[67]

> ## In summary: amputations of the index finger
>
> In summary for the index finger, it appears that preservation of range of motion is more important that salvaging length. A stiff index will be bypassed for the long finger and may hamper remaining hand function, whereas preservation of the proximal phalanx appears to be beneficial for hand function when compared with a ray amputation. We would still recommend that index ray amputation be performed as a secondary procedure, so the patient can be counseled about the risks of dysesthesia and loss of hand strength before undergoing the procedure.

Long Finger Amputation

The long finger provides the most finger flexion force when tested individually,[68,69] making it critical in power grip, but this digit is also key in precision pinch. Patients are easily able to substitute this digit for terminal and subterminal pinch following the loss of the index finger. The long finger's lack of the first dorsal interosseous muscle reduces its specialization when performing pinch functions. Transfer of the first dorsal interosseous to the insertion of the second dorsal interosseous has been suggested following first ray resection; however, studies have shown that this does not significantly increase pinch strength[70] and can lead to an intrinsic plus deformity in the long finger.[65,71]

Ring Finger Amputation

The ring finger has less strength than either the index or long. It is also rarely used for precision

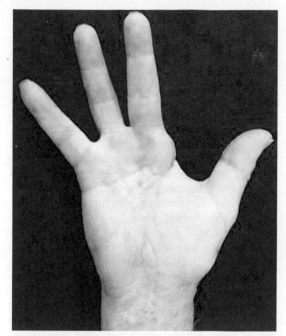

Fig. 8. Example of a functional index ray amputation. Notice preservation of good first web space at expense of loss of hand width.

pinch or grip. As an individual digit, Tubiana and Mackin[12] believed the ring finger's loss leaves the least functional deficit in the hand. When this finger is combined with the small as a functional unit, however, it can provide for adequate power grip and replace the index and long for pinch maneuvers should both digits be lost.

Central ray deletion, or loss of both ring and long fingers, may produce scissoring of the remaining border digits secondary to transverse metacarpal ligament instability and compromised interosseous function. Three-point chuck pinch is compromised, as is hand competence, because small objects may fall through the central defect.[72–74] Acute central ray resection with repair of the transverse metacarpal ligament may still result in scissoring of the neighboring digits, inadequate closure of the gap, and loss of abduction of the small ray.[73,75,76] In cases of central digital loss, a ray transposition may alleviate hand incompetence and reduce scissoring of the digits (**Fig. 9**). Results of strength testing following ray transposition for central digital loss have found an average decrease in grip and pinch strength of 20%, with larger decreases in function being seen for index to long transfer when compared with small to ring transfers. Loss of motion was only 9% following transfer.[75] A recent study comparing immediate/early to delayed fifth ray transposition following severe ring finger injury demonstrated superior grip, key pinch, pronation and supination strength, and fifth MCP joint range of motion among the immediate/early transposition group.[77] Although ray amputation may be indicated in cases of central digital loss,

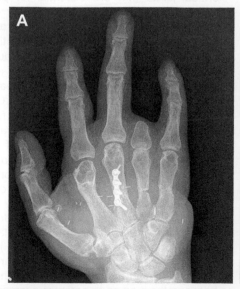
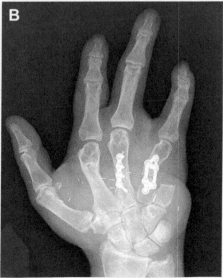

Fig. 9. AP radiographs of a 38-year-old steel worker's hand following a ring finger amputation and partial hand avulsion through the metacarpal shafts (*A*). Patient complained of hand incompetence. To reduce hand incompetence but maintain hand width, a small finger to ring finger transposition was performed. AP radiograph following transfer (*B*).

and may lead to ultimately better functional outcomes, it seems most prudent to perform this procedure after lengthy discussion has been carried out with the patient regarding his or her needs with regard to hand strength and motion.

Small Finger Amputation

Following the thumb, Tubiana and Mackin[12] believed the fifth finger provided the greatest functional value to hand function. The small finger has the least strength in flexion, but the small finger CMC joint can contribute up to 25° of flexion to the fingers overall range of motion. This allows the fifth ray to press objects and tools into the palm with a cupping motion that aids in digital palmar grip. Furthermore, the hypothenar muscles not only stabilize the metacarpal but also augment flexion of the first phalanx of the small finger. Stabilization is also added by the hypothenar muscles, which augment the flexion of the first phalanx of the small finger. In addition, the small finger's abduction capabilities significantly enhance span grasp.

In summary: amputations of the long, ring, and small fingers

The small finger can provide a great functional benefit in the hand due to the motion provided by its mobile CMC joint and the attachments of the hypothenar muscles. The middle finger has the greatest capacity for generating power grip due its size and muscle cross-sectional area. It also easily substitutes for the index finger to restore precision pinch. The ring finger when preserved with the small or long finger can contribute to chuck grip and power grasp; however, by itself the finger lacks the strength of the long finger, and the motion of the small finger. Finally, central amputations can have a detrimental effect on finger motion and hand competence. Although ray amputation can improve hand competence, it may have a negative impact on hand strength. We would recommend that formal ray amputation always be reserved as a secondary procedure.

Single-digit and multiple-digit loss

For the most part, a single-digit amputation, with the exception of the thumb, does not result in the loss of essential hand function. In a cohort of 183 surgeons that had sustained partial or total digital amputations, only 4 surgeons were unable to operate following their injuries.[20] Of this cohort, 15 surgeons (1 of whom is a hand surgeon) had a thumb amputation through the metacarpal or MP joint level, yet they were able to continue operating in their surgical practice. The investigators concluded that perhaps patient motivation is the greatest predictor of functional outcome rather than the specific digit or number of digits involved.[20] This conclusion may not translate to individuals conducting heavy manual labor.

Although single-digit amputation can be overcome by the motivated patient, multiple-digit amputation remains a challenging problem. Unfortunately, in the mutilated hand, multiple digital loss is frequent, particularly when a crush or avulsion component exist and prevents replantation. Preservation of the thumb and a single digit allows for some prehensile grasp, but for optimal function the reconstruction of an additional digit is recommended.[32,78–81] The thumb and 2 digits allows for the possibility of chuck pinch, which is stronger than subterminal pinch. The use of a third digit confers lateral stability in power pinch. A third digit also allows the patient to perform hook grip and power grasp. Finally, with a third digit, span grasp is now possible because functional palmar space is increased allowing for the grasp of larger objects.[32,78–81]

With severe multidigit amputation injuries with soft tissue loss, a staged approach is necessary for reconstruction. First, stable, soft tissue coverage is required as the "set up" for a later toe-to-thumb transfer.[81] Similarly, if a prosthetic is planned, adequate soft tissue, will be key in preserving length or protecting critical joints that are essential for prosthesis fitting.[81]

In injuries in which there is loss of all fingers but sparing of the thumb, reconstructive goals should attempt to maintain a useful thumb web space and an opposable ulnar post of adequate length. Additional digits may be created with microvascular toe transfer.[32,79,80,82,83] Other options include the transfer of remaining functional digits to more useful positions. Transferring salvageable digits to the ulnar side of the hand maintains the width of the palm, and allows for power grasp and the incorporation of pinch.[29,30,32] The radial placement of reconstructed digits is more cosmetically pleasing but fails to take advantage of the added power provided by intact hypothenar musculature and the motion provided by the fifth CMC joint. Wei and Colony[32] recommend that toes are placed next to remaining mobile fingers or in the interval between them so as to optimize cosmesis, coordinated digital movement, and smooth oppositional contact. However, there is some debate on ideal toe placement in a mutilated hand.[31,83,84] The decision may depend on hand dominance, with some recommending placing the toes in the index-middle position for fine pinching in the dominant hand, while toe placement in the nondominant hand to replace the fourth to fifth to produce a larger span.[81]

In cases in which there has been loss of all digits including the thumb, microvascular reconstruction of the thumb is required with the additional creation of a stable ulnar post. The previous practice of constructing a cleft hand (the Krukenberg procedure) has been shown to provide little benefit for hand function. It often has no effective prehension or grasp and does not adequately compare with the results obtainable with microsurgical reconstruction.[32,79,80,82,83] A recent algorithm for reconstruction following mutilating hand injuries recommends an ipsilateral great toe and a contralateral tandem toe transfer in the middle and ring positions for webspace preservation.[81]

Webspace Preservation

First web contracture is a common issue after trauma, due to direct trauma to the thenar and adductor muscles or because of prolonged immobilization. First web space contracture limits thumb function and prehensile activities. The first web space may be considered a triangle with the TMC joint at the apex and the thumb and index metacarpals forming 2 limbs of the triangle. Even minimal degrees of contracture at the apex will translate into severe limitations on the patient's ability to grasp and accommodate large objects, detracting from hand function.[85] It is best to prevent webspace contracture by recognizing and addressing potential causes early. It is a multifactorial problem that can arise from linear wounds in the webspace, hematoma, compartment syndrome, and adhesions secondary to local trauma. In the context of thumb amputation, first web contracture can be rapidly progressive. Del Pinal[3] recommends that early toe-to-thumb transfer followed by night splinting to prevent contracture of the thenar musculature. With a multidigit amputation scenario, resection of the second ray will address the contracted web and the index may even be appropriate for thumb reconstruction or contribute to soft tissue coverage for a thumb reconstruction.

Biomechanical Implications of Fusions

Partial or complete digit amputation are commonly cited as having poor functional outcomes after replantation or revascularization, especially in the case of complete amputation or when there is damage to the interphalangeal joints or MCP joints.[86,87] Concern regarding poor function with joint involvement leads many investigators to recommend revision amputation, as the severity of the trauma precludes any anatomic restoration of the joint surface.[88] However, a large number of patients desire the replantation of their amputated fingers. These situations may require immediate fusion when the digit is shortened during replantation. Unfortunately, change in a single joint has implications on the balance of the entire digit, and the biomechanics of the hand. The impact of arthrodesis and alternatives for joint restoration will be discussed for DIP, PIP, and MCP joints.

Finger Fusion

Distal interphalangeal joint fusions are generally well tolerated. Fifteen percent of intrinsic digital flexion occurs at the DIP joint, yet this translates into only 3% to the overall flexion arc of the finger.[89] Arthrodesis at this level imparts the least detriment to hand function with the relatively minor impact on finger arc of motion. Recent mechanical testing has shown that after simulated DIP fusion of the index and middle fingers, there is a 20% to 25% reduction in grip strength when compared with prefusion values. The decreased grip strength may be related to the quadriga effect, which limits terminal profundus flexion. It has been suggested that fusion in a more flexed position creates additional slack in the profundus tendon, decreasing the loss of grip strength.[90] A mild amount of flexion is recommended for optimal prehension.[91] When simulated, flexion of the index finger to 20 compared with fully extended fusion angle resulted in improved grip strength and dexterity but did not result in functional benefits when performed in the long finger.[92] The benefit of a flexed DIP joint position has not been validated in any comparative clinically studies and is an area for further study. For most individuals, with the exception of musicians, arthrodesis is preferred over arthroplasty at the DIP level.

Littler and Thompson[93] described the PIP joint as the, "functional locus of finger function." PIP joint impairment can adversely affect the entire hand. The PIP joint produces 85% of intrinsic digital flexion and contributes 20% to the overall arc of finger motion; however, a full range of PIP joint motion is not essential for hand function. An arc extending from 45 to 90° can provide relatively normal function.[94,95] The hand can compensate for a mild PIP joint flexor contracture through hyperextension of the MP joint. MCP hyperextension allows the finger to move out of the plane of the palm when attempting to lay the hand flat, performing precision tasks or when placing objects into the palm.[96]

When PIP joint fusion is necessary during reconstruction, its adverse effects on hand function will depend on the finger fused. Index finger PIP fusion is generally well tolerated, and has been shown to result in fewer complications over arthroplasty.[97] Index profundus function is relatively independent of the remaining 3 fingers and does not impose a significant quadriga effect on the other fingers during power grasp; however, long finger PIP fusion has been demonstrated to decrease excursion of all profundus tendons and produces a reduction in grip strength. PIP fusions will restrict profundus excursion to a greater extent than DIP or MP fusion.[65,98,99] In a study by Lista and colleagues,[98] a significant decrease in grip strength occurred when the PIP joints of the index and small fingers were fixed at less than 45° and when the long and the ring were fused in a position of less than 60° of flexion. Lower-demand activities of daily living were not significantly impacted in a simulated PIP joint arthrodesis study with flexion of 40°,[96] irrespective of the digit; however, subjects reported more difficulty with higher-demand activities. In the index, the workspace of the digit in the sagittal plane was optimal with simulated fusion of 40 to 50°.[100] Like the DIP joint, there are few clinical data comparing optimal fusion angles for each finger; this is an area for further study.

In cases in which both the MP and PIP joints are injured, MP joint salvage through arthroplasty or other measures is the priority over PIP joint arthroplasty. Although the resultant quadriga effect and grip strength reduction of PIP joint fusion should be expected, prehension can be maintained as long as the thumb or border digit is capable of opposition. The surgeon also should be aware that fusion of 2 sequential joints increase stress at the next proximal joint, due to an increase length in the lever arm working across the joint. This may accelerate the degeneration of adjacent joints if they are also injured.

Delayed reconstruction of the proximal interphalangeal joint in the setting of posttraumatic joint destruction is a challenging problem. In patients wishing to maintain some range of motion, arthroplasty is performed using a silicone implant, surface replacement arthroplasty, or vascularized toe-joint transfer. A systematic review comparing posttraumatic PIPJ arthroplasty using vascularized toe-joint transfer, silicone arthroplasty, or pyrocarbon arthroplasty found that the mean PIP joint active arcs of motion were 37.9°, 44.11°, and 43.11°, respectively.[101] There are increasing reports of delayed surface replacement arthroplasty for cases of PIP joint trauma.[97,102] Classic teaching has suggested that index PIP joint arthrodesis is preferred over arthroplasty to provide stability for key pinch. Surface replacement arthroplasty, however, may provide adequate stability for index finger PIP arthroplasty. Index PIPJ arthrodesis and surface replacement arthroplasty both result in increased oppositional pinch. Arthroplasty maintained preoperative range of motion, whereas arthrodesis resulted in improved appositional pinch and decreased time to and risk of complication.[97] Other reports of pyrocarbon arthroplasty demonstrated no significant change in the PIPJ range of motion, but significantly increased average grip and pinch strengths.[103] Hemiarthroplasty with a pyrocarbon implant also can be used if the proximal middle phalanx joint surface has minimal injury Hemiarthroplasty has demonstrated reduced pain and improved patient-reported function and satisfaction; however, this did not result in improved range of PIPJ motion.[104]

The MP joint is the most important joint for hand function, contributing up to 77% of the total arc of finger flexion.[89,93,94,105] Unlike the ginglymoid IP joint, which functions like a sloppy hinge joint, the condyloid MCP joint is diarthrodial, allowing for flexion-extension, abduction-adduction, and some rotation.[105–108] Most prehension grips require that the digits extend and abduct at the MP joint.[106,107] Precision pinch requires flexion, rotation, and ulnar deviation at the MP joint.[106,107] During pinch, the radial intrinsics and the collateral ligament to the index must resist the stress applied by the thumb. According to the American Medical Association's Guide to the Evaluation of Permanent Impairment, fusion of the MP joint results in a 45% impairment of the involved finger.[109] Some have suggested that a single stiff MP joint can impair the entire hand's function.[110] A full range of motion, however, is not required for daily hand function. Most activities of daily living require only 50% of normal joint motion.[106,111,112] MP motion of 35° within a functional range can lead to satisfactory function if the patient has a stable joint.[106] For an example of this, one need only think of our rheumatoid patients who are able to perform daily activities with fusions of the PIP and DIP joints but preservation or replacement of their MCP joints (Fig. 10).

Conventional algorithms recommend MCP arthrodesis for border digits in heavy laborers; however, surface replacement arthroplasty provides a motion-sparing alternative.[71,112,113] Acute MCP joint pyrocarbon arthroplasty has demonstrated restoration of MCP joint motion averaging 56°. A recent report looking at acute MCP arthroplasty in cases of trauma have found

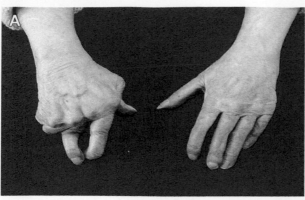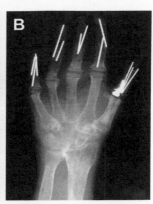

Fig. 10. Experience with patients with severe rheumatoid arthritis has shown us that preservation of MCP motion, through arthroplasty and PIP and DIP fusion, still allows for reasonable hand function. (*A*) Reconstructed left hand and unreconstructed hand in a 65-year-old woman with destructive rheumatoid arthritis. Patient is functional despite motion on left hand, which is limited to MCP joints. (*B*) AP radiograph of hand.

that this technique was capable of restoring grip, as well as appositional and oppositional pinch (28 kg, 11 kg, and 9 kg, respectively). No cases required joint revision. The investigators concluded that this is a safe technique in open MCP joint injuries with unsalvageable articular surfaces.[113] We have considered this to be one of the greatest advancements for the treatment of our acute trauma patients and has allowed the preservation of joint motion, which subsequently has improved the rehabilitation of tendon injuries as well as neighboring joint motion (**Fig. 11**).

Acute wrist fusion

Moving more proximal in the hand, immediate wrist fusions following trauma are rare, and usually are required following certain types of trauma, such as ballistic or punch-press type injuries. A stable wrist is the foundation for power grasp and prevents the dissipation of finger flexion and extension forces as tendons pass over the carpus. A stable wrist also allows for initiation of early hand and finger therapy.

Although the normal wrist has an average flexion-extension arc of 133°, the minimal amount of motion required for functional wrist motion has been debated. Reported functional palmar flexion ranges from 5 to 40° and functional dorsiflexion ranges from 30 to 40°. Minimal amounts of wrist deviation are required and have been reported to be 10° of radial deviation and 30° of ulnar deviation.[114–116] More recently, the importance of the "dart thrower's" motion has been highlighted as one of the functional axis of the wrist and reported to be 22° along the radially extended to ulnarly flexed positions.[117]

Limited carpal fusions consist of intercarpal fusions and radiocarpal fusions, which preserve

some wrist range of motion through the midcarpal joint. Mechanical studies by Meyerdierks and colleagues[118] show that fusions that cross the radiocarpal joint produce the greatest loss of motion. On average radiolunate, radioscapholunate (RSL), and radioscaphoid fusions decrease the flexion-extension arc by greater than 50%. To improve on this motion, recent studies have recommended removal of the distal pole of the scaphoid in cases of radioscapholunate fusions, thus unlocking the capitate and allowing for midcarpal motion. In the laboratory setting, distal pole resection of the scaphoid has produced flexion-extension arcs that are equivalent to normal wrist motion.[119] Calfee and colleagues[120] demonstrated a 38% and 43% reduction in flexion-extension and radial-ulnar deviation arcs of motion, respectively, following cadaveric RSL fusion; however, the remaining motion was maximally preserved along the dart thrower's plane through preservation of motion through the midcarpal joint. This biomechanical study also identified increased lunotriquetral, scaphotrapezial, scaphocapitate, and triquetrohamate motion, which may explain later development of midcarpalarthritis.[120]

Fusions that cross the midcarpal joint result in the next largest loss of wrist motion. Scaphocapitolunate and capitolunate fusion can produce a 35% loss of the flexion and extension arcs and up to a 31% loss of radial and ulnar deviation. Scaphotrapezial-trapezoid fusion produces a 23% decrease in the flexion-extension arc and 31% decrease in radial and ulnar deviation, whereas scaphocapitate fusion results in a 19% loss in the flexion-extension arc and a 19% loss in radial and ulnar deviation. Inclusion of the lunate within partial wrist fusions was found to nearly double the resultant loss of wrist motion when

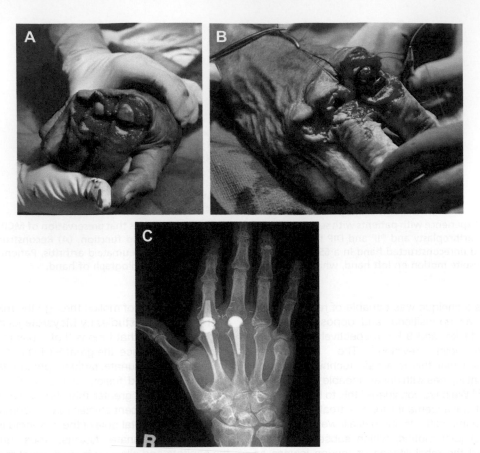

Fig. 11. An 84-year-old man who injured his hand with a table saw (A). The extensor tendons and joint surfaces of the MCP joint are injured. The wound was thoroughly debrided and a decision was made to reconstruct the joint with an immediate MCP joint arthroplasty and extensor tendon repair (B). (C) AP radiographs at 1 year. We feel this type of reconstruction provides benefits over delayed reconstruction by allowing immediate motion and improved tendon rehabilitation.

compared with fusions that did not include the lunate.[118] Fusion within the same carpal row tends to have a minimal effect on overall wrist motion, with average loss of only 12% of the flexion and extension arc. More recently, cadaveric study of 2-bone, 3-bone, and 4-bone partial wrist fusions found 4-bone fusion resulted in decreased palmar flexion, whereas all partial fusions resulted in decreased extension and the radial-extended position. There was no difference in dart thrower's motion between the different combinations of partial wrist fusion.[121]

The choice for total wrist fusion following mutilating hand trouma must be carefully considered; however, in cases of substantial carpal loss or destruction, this procedure may be the only option. The surgeon must keep in mind that removal of all wrist motion results in the loss of the beneficial effect of tenodesis for any subsequent tendon transfer. In addition, wrist dorsiflexion is important

for pushing off, rising from a chair, and power grasp.

Wrist fusion can have a negative impact on MP motion and thumb motion, which is likely attributable to extensor tendon adhesions over hardware.[122] A 25% decrease in grip strength may be seen, whereas key pinch, subterminal pinch, and directional grip are better maintained at approximately 85% of the normal side.[122,123] The ideal position for maximal preservation of power grip has been shown at 15° of extension and 15° of ulnar deviation.[124] Patient reports of postwrist arthrodesis function show the capacity to complete 85% of the activities of daily living as compared with preoperative status.[125] Patients were able to use a screwdriver and perform perineal care. Overall, skills that presented the most difficulty were those that required significant wrist flexion in a small space, where compensatory movements by the shoulder and elbow are eliminated. More recently, long-term follow-up on patients with bilateral total wrist arthrodesis demonstrated significant improvement in grip and pain levels. In addition, 93% of patients were satisfied with surgical outcomes and adapted to achieve a satisfactory level of extremity function.[126] Newer designs of wrist replacements may allow for reconstruction of the severely traumatized wrist, however at this time point most wrist arthroplasties are recommended for individuals who have low lifting demands.[127] Free-vascularized joint transfer for reconstruction of the traumatized radius to reconstruct the scaphoid fossa or lunate fossa (+/− sigmoid notch) has also been described.[128] Medium-term results demonstrated reduced patient-reported pain and DASH scores with maintenance of a limited range of motion; however, long-term results have not yet been reported.

In severely mutilating trauma, the preservation of wrist mobility imparts some function to a forearm stump with the addition of prosthesis. Modern prosthetic techniques allow the incorporation of the prosthesis to the wrist so that proximal straps and attachment to the elbow are unnecessary. Preservation of wrist motion also eliminates the need to incorporate a wrist articulation into the prosthetic unit.[8,19,129] In addition, preservation of the distal radio-ulnar joint (DRUJ) further improves function, because 50% of forearm rotation can be transferred into the prosthesis.[130] In addition, stable soft tissue coverage is critical for preserving proximal stump length and critical joints. When replantation is not possible, the use of fillet flaps from the amputated part or free tissue transfer aid in prosthetic fitting and comfort.[131,132]

Tendon loss Mutilating hand trauma has varying degrees of tendon involvement; tendons may be divided, avulsed, or have large segmental gaps that prohibit immediate repair. It is important to understand how tendon loss affects hand function.

Extensor tendons There are many factors that contribute to poor outcomes following extensor tendon injuries; these include[133–135] the superficial position of the extensor tendons, their complex architecture, and paucity of surrounding subcutaneous tissue.[135,136] As a consequence, it is common for patients to develop postoperative adhesions, which limit flexion and produce extensor lags and subsequent functional deficits.[137] It has been shown that injuries in the distal zones (1 through 5) result in poorer outcomes and greater postoperative extension deficits. Extensor tendon injuries also carry a significantly worse prognosis when associated with underlying fractures.[21,135]

The extensor mechanism has a smaller excursion than the flexor system, particularly about the PIP joint where excursion is between 2 and 5 mm.[138,139] This leaves little margin for adherence or shortening if PIP joint motion is to be maintained. In the instance of significant shortening with repair, the extensor mechanism has less ability to compensate because of the interconnections between the intrinsic and extrinsic mechanisms. If significant shortening results from a primary repair with intact lateral bands and oblique retinacular ligament, one can opt to leave the central extensor mechanism unrepaired. This may avoid flexion loss, without producing a PIP or DIP extension lag. In the setting of segmental loss in zone 2 or 4 injuries, distally based proximal tendon flaps can be used to reconstruct a defect of up to 5 mm and 10 mm, respectively.[140] Loss of long extensor function can destabilize the MP joint, however, resulting in a loss of active finger abduction-adduction.[141] Further biomechanical studies are required to determine the absolute requirements for functional finger extension.

Restoration of full-finger extension is maximized when intrinsic function can be preserved; unfortunately, in mutilating hand injuries, intrinsic function may likely be compromised after crush injuries and metacarpal fractures with direct muscle trauma. Additionally, intrinsics may lose biomechanical advantage in the setting of metacarpal shortening or fracture angulation beyond 30°, which results in a shortening of intrinsic muscle fiber length,[129] and the potential excursion of the intrinsic tendon.[39] With metacarpal malreduction or shortening, starting muscle tension is also decreased. These factors decrease intrinsic tendon excursion and joint motion.[129,142] This loss of intrinsic function emphases the need for preservation of metacarpal length and the anatomic reductions of fractures in cases of significant hand trauma. Stable fixation of bony trauma will also facilitate earlier extensor tendon rehabilitation, reducing the risk of tendon adhesion.[140]

Extensor tendon injuries proximal to the junctura may produce less postinjury deficits. Quaba and colleagues[143] examined 9 patients who lost finger extensors in zones 6 and 7. In this study, no attempt was made to reconstruct the tendons, but soft tissue coverage was provided to all defects. Surprisingly, in long-term follow-up, there was only a 26% decrease in total active finger motion, mainly affecting MP joints. With intact intrinsic function, DIP and PIP extension was preserved and active motion at the MP joint was only 60% of normal. Despite this deficit, 90% of patients were satisfied with hand function, noting difficulty with tying knots and unscrewing lids. When MP joint motion is limited, intact thumb abduction and extension are critical to bring the thumb out of the palm for prehension of objects with a moderately flexed posture of the digits. The loss of the central extensors decreases power grip by approximately 30%, whereas the loss of wrist extensors results in a 50% reduction in grip strength.[141,143]

Flexor tendons Injury to the profundus tendon can impair function of the individual digit as well as overall composite grip. DIP joint flexion is absent without profundus function and this will interfere with subterminal and terminal pinch. If the injured profundus tendon becomes adherent to the sublimis tendon or underlying metacarpal fracture callus, it may tether the profundus tendons of adjacent uninjured fingers, preventing full digitopalmar grip.[15,138] This linkage of the profundus tendons has classically been described as the *quadriga effect*, and typically only applies to the long through small fingers, because of their common muscle belly, but can extend to the index finger if heavy synovium at the level of the carpal tunnel links the index to the other 3 profundus tendons.[144] In addition, retraction of the profundus tendon, following more proximal amputations may result in shortening and eventual contracture of the corresponding lumbrical. During flexion, contraction of the profundus muscle belly places stretch on the shortened lumbrical, which results in paradoxic extension of the PIP joint, termed the *lumbrical plus deformity*. This deformity can be managed with division of the lumbrical or suturing the proximal cut profundus tendon to the flexor sheath in a relaxed position.[15,145]

Power grip and forceful pinch are still possible with superficialis loss; however, loss of the superficialis with preservation of the profundus tendon can create a phenomenon called *recurvatum*, in which the PIP joint is hyperextended. In exaggerated cases, this may produce delayed finger flexion. Recurvatum can be avoided by leaving the portion of the superficialis distal to the chiasm.[15] With loss of both profundus and superficialis tendons but intact intrinsic function, flexion of the MP joint to 45° may be possible.

With multiple digital amputations, retraction of the flexor mechanism can lead to lumbrical migration into the carpal tunnel with subsequent symptomatic median nerve compression.[8,146] These patients may not present with classic digital paresthesias if there has been significant digital soft tissue loss. Rather patients may complain of generalized pain within the wrist and palm, which may be exacerbated by the standard provocative maneuvers. Carpal tunnel release should be pursued in such instances.

A2 and A4 pulley preservation is critical and bowstringing will ensue if either is divided.[147–150] The A2 and A4 pulleys are located over the bony shafts of the proximal and middle phalanx. This anatomic configuration prevents the bowstringing that occurs with joint flexion and the bowstringing that can occur over the phalanx shaft. Palmar plate pulleys (A1, A3, and A5) have a variable relationship to the joint axis depending on joint position, and restrain only the joint-type of bowstringing. They also narrow up to 50% with finger flexion, which reduces their efficiency. Cruciate pulleys have little effect on restraining bowstringing.[148,150] Some investigators have described completely venting the A4 pulley to facilitate tendon repair and allow for tendon gliding and showed no increase in bowstringing. In addition, venting of the A4 pulley resulted in less force required for flexion than with an intact or repaired pulley.[151,152] Thus, in circumstances in which the A4 must be sacrificed for repair or gliding purposes, repair may not be necessary. If bowstringing does occur, it will result in an increase in the flexion moment arm at the PIP and MP joints. A longer moment arm disrupts the balance of joint flexion and extension forces; subsequently, with a longer flexor moment arm the flexor forces will overcome the extension forces, resulting in a flexion deformity. A longer moment arm also means the tendon must move through a longer distance to obtain the same motion at the joint, decreasing mechanical efficiency. As in the quadriga effect, grip strength will be decreased with bowstringing because full excursion is now limited.[150]

Decision for hand transplantation The decision for hand transplantation following mutilating hand trauma is rare but sometimes the injuries are beyond the scope of repair. The ideal patient for consideration of hand transplantation is a patient with bilateral distal forearm amputations. Although these patients present in times of military conflict, bilateral amputees eligible for bilateral hand transplantation in civilian trauma within the United States are few in number. Many of the patients evaluated in our institutions are upper and lower limb amputees as the result of sepsis rather than direct hand trauma. Regardless, if it is deemed appropriate to proceed with hand transplantation, most centers require a 6-month to 12-month period for trialing bilateral prosthesis. In preparation for transplantation, one should consider preservation of the tendon muscle junction, as this is difficult to reconstruct during the transplantation procedure. In addition, preservation of nerve length should be considered at the time of initial amputation. More proximal resection of the nerve stumps has not been clearly shown to prevent pain or neuroma formation and will only lengthen recovery of intrinsic function should the patient decide to proceed with hand transplantation.

FUTURE DIRECTIONS

Future research should focus on outcomes in this patient population. The outcomes of acute post-traumatic arthroplasty need to be further examined along with newer options for fusions and partial joint replacement. Advancements in microsurgery continue to allow for restoration of bone and potentially cartilage.[153,154] Long-term prospective and cross-sectional data of these patients would help the surgeon to better understand the downstream implications of amputation versus salvage attempts.

SUMMARY

Surgeons managing mutilating hand injures are faced with difficult decisions between attempting to salvage remaining or injured digits or proceeding to amputation and fusion. With a basic understanding of hand biomechanics, the surgeon may more accurately assess what motion and function can best be salvaged. By understanding how amputation, fusion, and tendon loss affect postoperative hand motion, the surgeon can better focus his or her reconstructive efforts to achieve the highest functional outcome for the patient.

REFERENCES

1. Moran SL, Berger RA. Biomechanics and hand trauma: what you need. Hand Clin 2003;19:17–31.
2. Campbell DA, Kay SP. The hand injury severity scoring system. J Hand Surg Br 1996;21:295–8.
3. del Pinal F. Severe mutilating injuries to the hand: guidelines for organizing the chaos. J Plast Reconstr Aesthet Surg 2007;60:816–27.
4. German G, Sherman R, Levin LS. Decisionmaking in reconstructive surgery (upper extremity). Berlin: Springer; 2000.
5. Slauterbeck JR, Britton C, Moneim MS, et al. Mangled extremity severity score: an accurate guide to treatment of the severely injured upper extremity. J Orthop Trauma 1994;8:282–5.
6. Tomaino MM. Treatment of composite tissue loss following hand and forearm trauma. Hand Clin 1999;15:319–33, ix.
7. Weinzweig J, Weinzweig N. The "Tic-Tac-Toe" classification system for mutilating injuries of the hand. Plast Reconstr Surg 1997;100:1200–11.
8. Burkhalter W. Mutilating injuries of the hand. Hand Clin 1986;2:45–68.
9. Hentz Vr CR, editor. The philosophy of salvage and repair for acute hand injuries. St Louis (MO): Mosby; 1979.
10. Entin MA. Salvaging the basic hand. Surg Clin North Am 1968;48:1062–81.
11. Moberg E. Reconstructive hand surgery in tetraplegia, stroke, and cerebral palsy: basic concepts in physiology and neurology. J Hand Surg Am 1976; 1:29–34.
12. Tubiana R, Thomine J, Mackin E, editors. Movements of the hand and wrist. St Louis (MO): Mosby; 1996.
13. Rabischong P. Les problemes fondamentaux du retablissment de la prehension. Ann Chir 1971; 25:927.
14. Duparc J, Alnot J-Y, May P. Single digit amputations. In: Campbell DA, Gosset J, editors. Mutilating injuries of the hand. Edinburga: Churchill Livingstone; 1979. p. 37–44.
15. Smith P. Lister's the hand. London: Churchill Livingstone; 2002.
16. Michon J. Complex hand injuries: surgical planning. In: Tubiana R, editor. The hand, vol. 2. Philadelphia: WB Saunders; 1985. p. 196–213.
17. Arellano AO, Wegener EE, Freeland AE. Mutilating injuries to the hand: early amputation or repair and reconstruction. Orthopedics 1999;22:683–4.
18. Beasley RW, DG. Upper limb amputations and prostheses. In: Aston SJ, BR, Thorne CHM, editors. Philadelphia: Lippincott-Raven; 1997. p. 1009–20.
19. Brown PW. Sacrifice of the unsatisfactory hand. J Hand Surg Am 1979;4:417–23.
20. Brown PW. Less than ten: surgeons with amputated fingers. J Hand Surg Am 1982;7:31–7.
21. Duncan RW, Freeland AE, Jabaley ME, et al. Open hand fractures: an analysis of the recovery of active motion and of complications. J Hand Surg Am 1993;18:387–94.
22. McCormack RM. Primary reconstruction in acute hand injuries. Surg Clin North Am 1960;40:337–43.
23. Brooks D, Buntic RF, Taylor C. Use of the venous flap for salvage of difficult ring avulsion injuries. Microsurgery 2008;28:397–402.
24. Breahna A, Siddiqui A, Fitzgerald O'Connor E, et al. Replantation of digits: a review of predictive factors for survival. J Hand Surg Eur Vol 2016. [Epub ahead of print].
25. Fufa D, Calfee R, Wall L, et al. Digit replantation: experience of two U.S. academic level-I trauma centers. J Bone Joint Surg Am 2013;95:2127–34.
26. Huang D, Wang HG, Wu WZ, et al. Functional and aesthetic results of immediate reconstruction of traumatic thumb defects by toe-to-thumb transplantation. Int Orthop 2011;35:543–7.
27. Sebastin SJ, Chung KC. A systematic review of the outcomes of replantation of distal digital amputation. Plast Reconstr Surg 2011;128:723–37.

28. Curtis RM. Opposition of the thumb. Orthop Clin North Am 1974;5:305–21.

29. Soucacos PN. Indications and selection for digital amputation and replantation. J Hand Surg Br 2001;26:572–81.

30. Soucacos PN, Beris AE, Malizos KN, et al. Transpositional microsurgery in multiple digital amputations. Microsurgery 1994;15:469–73.

31. Strickland JW. Thumb reconstruction. In: Green DP, editor. Operative hand surgery. 2nd edition. New York: Churchill Livingstone; 1988. p. 2175–262.

32. Wei FC, Colony LH. Microsurgical reconstruction of opposable digits in mutilating hand injuries. Clin Plast Surg 1989;16:491–504.

33. Napier JR. The form and function of the carpometacarpal joint of the thumb. J Anat 1955;89: 362–9.

34. Cooney WP 3rd, Chao EY. Biomechanical analysis of static forces in the thumb during hand function. J Bone Joint Surg Am 1977;59:27–36.

35. Cooney WP, Linscheid RL, An KN. Opposition of the thumb: an anatomic and biomechanical study of tendon transfers. J Hand Surg Am 1984; 9:777–86.

36. Imaeda T, An KN, Cooney WP 3rd. Functional anatomy and biomechanics of the thumb. Hand Clin 1992;8:9–15.

37. Napier JR. The attachments and function of the abductor pollicis brevis. J Anat 1952;86:335–41.

38. Cooney WP 3rd, Lucca MJ, Chao EY, et al. The kinesiology of the thumb trapeziometacarpal joint. J Bone Joint Surg Am 1981;63:1371–81.

39. Brand PW, Beach RB, Thompson DE. Relative tension and potential excursion of muscles in the forearm and hand. J Hand Surg Am 1981;6: 209–19.

40. Kaplan EB. Function and surgical anatomy of the hand. 2nd edition. Philadelphia: Lippincott; 1965. p. 158–62.

41. Dell'oca RL, Hentz VR. Thumb reconstruction. In: Goldwyn RM, Cohen MN, editors. The unfavorable result in plastic surgery. Philadelphia: Lippincott; 2001. p. 805–29.

42. Urbaniak JR. Thumb reconstruction by microsurgery. Instr Course Lect 1984;33:425–46.

43. Morrison WA. Thumb reconstruction: a review and philosophy of management. J Hand Surg Br 1992;17:383–90.

44. Morrison WA, O'Brien BM, MacLeod AM. Thumb reconstruction with a free neurovascular wraparound flap from the big toe. J Hand Surg Am 1980;5:575–83.

45. Matev IB. Reconstructive surgery of the thumb. Essex (England): Pilgrims Press; 1983.

46. Shin AY, Bishop AT, Berger RA. Microvascular reconstruction of the traumatized thumb. Hand Clin 1999;15:347–71.

47. Chung KC, Wei FC. An outcome study of thumb reconstruction using microvascular toe transfer. J Hand Surg Am 2000;25:651–8.

48. Lee KS, Park JW, Chung WK. Thumb reconstruction with a wraparound free flap according to the level of amputation. J Hand Surg Am 2000;25: 644–50.

49. Kotkansalo T, Vilkki S, Elo P, et al. Long-term functional results of microvascular toe-to-thumb reconstruction. J Hand Surg Eur Vol 2011;36:194–204.

50. Bosch M, Granell F, Faig-Marti J, et al. First metacarpal lengthening following traumatic amputation of the thumb: long-term follow-up. Chir Main 2004;23:284–8.

51. Leung PC. Thumb reconstruction using second-toe transfer. Hand 1983;15:15–21.

52. Bunnell S. Opposition of the thumb. J Bone Joint Surg 1938;20:269–84.

53. Duymaz A, Karabekmez FE, Zhao C, et al. Tendon transfer for the restoration of thumb opposition: the effects of friction and pulley location. Plast Reconstr Surg 2013;132:604–9.

54. Katarincic JA. Thumb kinematics and their relevance to function. Hand Clin 2001;17:169–74.

55. Bettinger PC, Berger RA. Functional ligamentous anatomy of the trapezium and trapeziometacarpal joint (gross and arthroscopic). Hand Clin 2001;17: 151–68, vii.

56. Bettinger PC, Linscheid RL, Berger RA, et al. An anatomic study of the stabilizing ligaments of the trapezium and trapeziometacarpal joint. J Hand Surg Am 1999;24:786–98.

57. Bravo CJ, Horton T, Moran SL, et al. Traumatized index finger pollicization for thumb reconstruction. J Hand Surg Am 2008;33:257–62.

58. Yu G, Xu HY, Lei HY, et al. Combined index finger pollicization with an anterolateral thigh flap for thumb reconstruction. Chin J Traumatol 2014;17:354–7.

59. Ishida O, Taniguchi Y, Sunagawa T, et al. Pollicization of the index finger for traumatic thumb amputation. Plast Reconstr Surg 2006;117:909–14.

60. Michon J, Merle M, Bouchon Y, et al. Functional comparison between pollicization and toe-to-hand transfer for thumb reconstruction. J Reconstr Microsurg 1984;1:103–12.

61. Buck-Gramcko D, Hoffman R, Neumann R. Hand trauma: a practical guide. New York: Theime; 1986. p. 60–73.

62. Campbell DA, Gosset J. Mutilating injuries of the hand. Edinburgh (United Kingdom): Churchill Livingstone; 1979. p. 37–44.

63. Buntic RF, Brooks D, Buncke GM. Index finger salvage with replantation and revascularization: revisiting conventional wisdom. Microsurgery 2008; 28:612–6.

64. White WL. Why I hate the index finger. Hand (N Y) 2010;5:461–5.

65. Murray JF, Carman W, MacKenzie JK. Transmetacarpal amputation of the index finger: a clinical assessment of hand strength and complications. J Hand Surg Am 1977;2:471–81.

66. Karle B, Wittemann M, Germann G. Functional outcome and quality of life after ray amputation versus amputation through the proximal phalanx of the index finger. Handchir Mikrochir Plast Chir 2002;34:30–5 [in German].

67. Wilkens SC, Claessen FM, Ogink PT, et al. Reoperation after combined injury of the index finger: repair versus immediate amputation. J Hand Surg Am 2016;41:436–40.e4.

68. Ejeskar A, Ortengren R. Isolated finger flexion force– a methodological study. Hand 1981;13:223–30.

69. Hazelton FT, Smidt GL, Flatt AE, et al. The influence of wrist position on the force produced by the finger flexors. J Biomech 1975;8:301–6.

70. Chase RA. The damaged index digit. A source of components to restore the crippled hand. J Bone Joint Surg Am 1968;50:1152–60.

71. Linscheid RL, Murray PM, Vidal MA, et al. Development of a surface replacement arthroplasty for proximal interphalangeal joints. J Hand Surg Am 1997;22:286–98.

72. Carroll RE. Transposition of the index finger to replace the middle finger. Clin Orthop 1959;15:27–34.

73. de Boer A, Robinson PH. Ray transposition by intercarpal osteotomy after loss of the fourth digit. J Hand Surg Am 1989;14:379–81.

74. Posner MA. Ray transposition for central digital loss. J Hand Surg Am 1979;4:242–57.

75. Colen L, Bunkis J, Gordon L, et al. Functional assessment of ray transfer for central digital loss. J Hand Surg Am 1985;10:232–7.

76. Steichen JB, Idler RS. Results of central ray resection without bony transposition. J Hand Surg Am 1986;11:466–74.

77. Sadek AF, Fouly EH, Hassan MY. Early versus delayed fourth ray amputation with fifth ray transposition for management of mutilating ring finger injuries. J Hand Surg Am 2015;40:1389–96.

78. Tsai TM, Jupiter JB, Wolff TW, et al. Reconstruction of severe transmetacarpal mutilating hand injuries by combined second and third toe transfer. J Hand Surg Am 1981;6:319–28.

79. Wei FC, Chen HC, Chuang CC, et al. Reconstruction of a hand, amputated at the metacarpophalangeal level, by means of combined second and third toes from each foot: a case report. J Hand Surg Am 1986;11:340–4.

80. Wei FC, Chen HC, Chuang CC, et al. Simultaneous multiple toe transfers in hand reconstruction. Plast Reconstr Surg 1988;81:366–77.

81. Ekwobi CC. Re: A novel technique for vacuum assisted closure device application in non-contiguous wounds, by A. Culliford IV, J. Spector, J. Levine, Journal of Plastic, Reconstructive & Aesthetic Surgery, 2007;60:99–100. J Plast Reconstr Aesthet Surg 2007;60:1268.

82. Gorsche TS, Wood MB. Mutilating corn-picker injuries of the hand. J Hand Surg Am 1988;13:423–7.

83. Wei FC, Colony LH, Chen HC, et al. Combined second and third toe transfer. Plast Reconstr Surg 1989;84:651–61.

84. Valauri FA, Buncke HJ. Thumb and finger reconstruction by toe-to-hand transfer. Hand Clin 1992;8:551–74.

85. Del Pinal F, Garcia-Bernal FJ, Delgado J. Is posttraumatic first web contracture avoidable? Prophylactic guidelines and treatment-oriented classification. Plast Reconstr Surg 2004;113:1855–60.

86. Pederson WC. Replantation. Plast Reconstr Surg 2001;107:823–41.

87. Medling BD, Bueno RA Jr, Russell RC, et al. Replantation outcomes. Clin Plast Surg 2007;34:177–85. vii-viii.

88. Sears ED, Chung KC. Replantation of finger avulsion injuries: a systematic review of survival and functional outcomes. J Hand Surg Am 2011;36:686–94.

89. Littler JW, Herndon JH, Thompson JS. Examination of the hand. In: Converse JM, Littler JW, editors. Reconstructive plastic surgery. vol. 6. Philadelphia: WB Saunders; 1977. p. 2973.

90. Morgan WJ, Schulz LA, Chang JL. The impact of simulated distal interphalangeal joint fusion on grip strength. Orthopedics 2000;23:239–41.

91. Tomaino MM. Distal interphalangeal joint arthrodesis with screw fixation: why and how. Hand Clin 2006;22:207–10.

92. Melamed E, Polatsch DB, Beldner S, et al. Simulated distal interphalangeal joint fusion of the index and middle fingers in 0 degrees and 20 degrees of flexion: a comparison of grip strength and dexterity. J Hand Surg Am 2014;39:1986–91.

93. Littler JW, Thompson JS. Surgical and functional anatomy. In: Bowers WH, editor. The interphalangeal joints. New York: Churchill Livingstone; 1987. p. 142.

94. Foucher G, Hoang P, Citron N, et al. Joint reconstruction following trauma: comparison of microsurgical transfer and conventional methods: a report of 61 cases. J Hand Surg Br 1986;11:388–93.

95. An KN, Chao EY, Cooney WP, et al. Forces in the normal and abnormal hand. J Orthop Res 1985;3:202–11.

96. Woodworth JA, McCullough MB, Grosland NM, et al. Impact of simulated proximal interphalangeal arthrodeses of all fingers on hand function. J Hand Surg Am 2006;31:940–6.

97. Vitale MA, Fruth KM, Rizzo M, et al. Prosthetic arthroplasty versus arthrodesis for osteoarthritis and

posttraumatic arthritis of the index finger proximal interphalangeal joint. J Hand Surg Am 2015;40: 1937–48.

98. Lista FR, Neu BR, Murray JF, et al. Profundus tendon blockage (the quadrigia syndrome) in the hand with a stiff finger. 43rd annual meeting of the American Society for Surgery of the Hand. Baltimore, September, 1988.

99. Neu BR, Murray JF, MacKenzie JK. Profundus tendon blockage: quadriga in finger amputations. J Hand Surg Am 1985;10:878–83.

100. Arauz PG, Sisto SA, Kao I. Assessment of workspace attributes under simulated index finger proximal interphalangeal arthrodesis. J Biomech Eng 2016;138(5):051005.

101. Squitieri L, Chung KC. A systematic review of outcomes and complications of vascularized toe joint transfer, silicone arthroplasty, and PyroCarbon arthroplasty for posttraumatic joint reconstruction of the finger. Plast Reconstr Surg 2008;121:1697–707.

102. Wagner ER, Luo TD, Houdek MT, et al. Revision proximal interphalangeal arthroplasty: an outcome analysis of 75 consecutive cases. J Hand Surg Am 2015;40:1949–55.e1.

103. Nunley RM, Boyer MI, Goldfarb CA. Pyrolytic carbon arthroplasty for posttraumatic arthritis of the proximal interphalangeal joint. J Hand Surg Am 2006;31:1468–74.

104. Pettersson K, Amilon A, Rizzo M. Pyrolytic carbon hemiarthroplasty in the management of proximal interphalangeal joint arthritis. J Hand Surg Am 2015;40:462–8.

105. Ellis PR, Tsai TM. Management of the traumatized joint of the finger. Clin Plast Surg 1989;16:457–73.

106. Beckenbaugh RD, Dobyns JH, Linscheid RL, et al. Review and analysis of silicone-rubber metacarpophalangeal implants. J Bone Joint Surg Am 1976; 58:483–7.

107. Flatt AE. Care of the rheumatoid hand. 4th edition. St Louis (MO): Mosby; 1983.

108. Krishnan J, Chipchase L. Passive axial rotation of the metacarpophalangeal joint. J Hand Surg Br 1997;22:270–3.

109. Association AM. Guides to the evaluation of permanent impairment. 2nd edition. Chicago: American Medical Association; 1984.

110. Hagert CG, Branemark PI, Albrektsson T, et al. Metacarpophalangeal joint replacement with osseointegrated endoprostheses. Scand J Plast Reconstr Surg 1986;20:207–18.

111. Doi K, Kuwata N, Kawai S. Alumina ceramic finger implants: a preliminary biomaterial and clinical evaluation. J Hand Surg Am 1984;9:740–9.

112. Lischeid RL, Beckenbaugh RD. Arthroplasty of the metacarpal phalangeal joint. In: Morrey BF, An K-N, editors. Reconstructive surgery of the joints. 2nd edition. New York: Churchill Livingstone; 1996. p. 287.

113. Houdek MT, Wagner ER, Rizzo M, et al. Metacarpophalangeal joint arthroplasty in the setting of trauma. J Hand Surg Am 2015;40:2416–20.

114. Palmer AK, Werner FW, Murphy D, et al. Functional wrist motion: a biomechanical study. J Hand Surg Am 1985;10:39–46.

115. Brumfield RH, Champoux JA. A biomechanical study of normal functional wrist motion. Clin Orthop Relat Res 1984;(187):23–5.

116. Ryu JY, Cooney WP 3rd, Askew LJ, et al. Functional ranges of motion of the wrist joint. J Hand Surg Am 1991;16:409–19.

117. Crisco JJ, Heard WM, Rich RR, et al. The mechanical axes of the wrist are oriented obliquely to the anatomical axes. J Bone Joint Surg Am 2011;93: 169–77.

118. Meyerdierks EM, Mosher JF, Werner FW. Limited wrist arthrodesis: a laboratory study. J Hand Surg Am 1987;12:526–9.

119. McCombe D, Ireland DC, McNab I. Distal scaphoid excision after radioscaphoid arthrodesis. J Hand Surg Am 2001;26:877–82.

120. Calfee RP, Leventhal EL, Wilkerson J, et al. Simulated radioscapholunate fusion alters carpal kinematics while preserving dart-thrower's motion. J Hand Surg Am 2008;33:503–10.

121. Got C, Vopat BG, Mansuripur PK, et al. The effects of partial carpal fusions on wrist range of motion. J Hand Surg Eur Vol 2015;41(5):479–83.

122. Field J, Herbert TJ, Prosser R. Total wrist fusion. A functional assessment. J Hand Surg Br 1996;21: 429–33.

123. Labosky DA, Waggy CA. Apparent weakness of median and ulnar motors in radial nerve palsy. J Hand Surg Am 1986;11:528–33.

124. Pryce JC. The wrist position between neutral and ulnar deviation that facilitates the maximum power grip strength. J Biomech 1980;13:505–11.

125. Weiss AC, Wiedeman G Jr, Quenzer D, et al. Upper extremity function after wrist arthrodesis. J Hand Surg Am 1995;20:813–7.

126. Wagner ER, Elhassan BT, Kakar S. Long-term functional outcomes after bilateral total wrist arthrodesis. J Hand Surg Am 2015;40:224–8.e1.

127. Kennedy CD, Huang JI. Prosthetic design in total wrist arthroplasty. Orthop Clin North Am 2016;47: 207–18.

128. Glatt H, Utesch D, Herbst M, et al. Mutagenicity experiments on L-cysteine and D-penicillamine using V79 cells as indicators and for metabolic activation. Mutat Res 1990;243:187–93.

129. Ali A, Hamman J, Mass DP. The biomechanical effects of angulated boxer's fractures. J Hand Surg Am 1999;24:835–44.

130. Wright TW, Hagen AD, Wood MB. Prosthetic usage in major upper extremity amputations. J Hand Surg Am 1995;20:619–22.

131. Oliveira IC, Barbosa RF, Ferreira PC, et al. The use of forearm free fillet flap in traumatic upper extremity amputations. Microsurgery 2009;29:8–15.

132. Flurry M, Melissinos EG, Livingston CK. Composite forearm free fillet flaps to preserve stump length following traumatic amputations of the upper extremity. Ann Plast Surg 2008;60:391–4.

133. Hauge MF. The results of tendon suture of the hand; a review of 500 patients. Acta Orthop Scand 1955;24:258–70.

134. Kelly AP Jr. Primary tendon repairs; a study of 789 consecutive tendon severances. J Bone Joint Surg Am 1959;41-A:581–98.

135. Verdan CE. Primary and secondary repair of flexor and extensor tendon injuries. In: Flynn JE, editor. Hand surgery. Baltimore (MD): Williams & Wilkins; 1966. p. 220–75.

136. Scheker LR, Langley SJ, Martin DL, et al. Primary extensor tendon reconstruction in dorsal hand defects requiring free flaps. J Hand Surg Br 1993; 18:568–75.

137. Hamada Y, Hibino N. The treatment of extensor lag of the middle finger following crushing-penetrating injuries of the metacarpophalangeal joint: case series. Hand (N Y) 2014;9:534–8.

138. Verdan C. Syndrome of the quadriga. Surg Clin North Am 1960;40:425–6.

139. De Voll JR, Saldana MJ. Excursion of finger extensor elements in zone III. Presented at the American Association for Hand Surgery; Toronto, Canada, 1988.

140. Lee SK, Dubey A, Kim BH, et al. A biomechanical study of extensor tendon repair methods: introduction to the running-interlocking horizontal mattress extensor tendon repair technique. J Hand Surg Am 2010;35:19–23.

141. Boyes JH. Bunnell's surgery of the hand. 5th edition. Philadelphia: Lippincott; 1967.

142. Elftman H. Biomechanics of muscle with particular application to studies of gait. J Bone Joint Surg Am 1966;48:363–77.

143. Quaba AA, Elliot D, Sommerlad BC. Long term hand function without long finger extensors: a clinical study. J Hand Surg Br 1988;13:66–71.

144. Fahrer M. In: Verdan C, editor. Tendon surgery of the hand. Edinburgh (United Kingdom): Churchill Livingstone; 1979. p. 17–24.

145. Louis DS, Jebson PJL, Graham TJ. Amputations. In: Green DP, Pederson W, editors. Green's operative hand surgery. 4th edition. New York: Churchill Livingstone; 1999. p. 48–75.

146. Cobb TK, An KN, Cooney WP, et al. Lumbrical muscle incursion into the carpal tunnel during finger flexion. J Hand Surg Br 1994;19:434–8.

147. Doyle JR, Blythe W. The finger flexor tendon sheath and pulleys: anatomy and reconstruction. In: Hunter JM, Schneider LH, editors. Symposium on tendon surgery in the hand. St Louis (MO): Mosby; 1975. p. 81–7.

148. Hume EL. Panel discussion: flexor tendon reconstruction. In: Hunter JM, Schneider LH, Mackin EJ, editors. Tendon surgery in the hand. St Louis (MO): Mosby; 1987. p. 658–62.

149. Idler RS. Anatomy and biomechanics of the digital flexor tendons. Hand Clin 1985;1:3–11.

150. Lin GT, Amadio PC, An KN, et al. Functional anatomy of the human digital flexor pulley system. J Hand Surg Am 1989;14:949–56.

151. Tang JB. Release of the A4 pulley to facilitate zone II flexor tendon repair. J Hand Surg Am 2014;39: 2300–7.

152. Franko OI, Lee NM, Finneran JJ, et al. Quantification of partial or complete A4 pulley release with FDP repair in cadaveric tendons. J Hand Surg Am 2011;36:439–45.

153. Higgins JP, Burger HK. Osteochondral flaps from the distal femur: expanding applications, harvest sites, and indications. J Reconstr Microsurg 2014; 30:483–90.

154. del Pinal F, Klausmeyer M, Moraleda E, et al. Vascularized graft from the metatarsal base for reconstructing major osteochondral distal radius defects. J Hand Surg Am 2013;38:1883–95.

Measuring Functional and Patient-Reported Outcomes After Treatment of Mutilating Hand Injuries
A Global Health Approach

Aviram M. Giladi, MD, MS*, Kavitha Ranganathan, MD,
Kevin C. Chung, MD, MS

KEYWORDS

- Patient-reported outcomes • Impairment and disability • DALY • Global health
- Mutilating upper extremity trauma

KEY POINTS

- Measuring outcomes after mutilating upper extremity trauma is key to understanding disability after these injuries, and holds major implications for addressing the global burden of extremity trauma.
- Patient-reported outcomes are necessary for understanding disability and associated quality of life after these injuries.
- Owing to the complexity and variability of massive upper extremity trauma, understanding outcomes requires a multimodal approach, along with improvements in data collection.
- Using outcomes measures to determine disability after extremity trauma is critical to understanding the value of associated surgical care delivery and resource use.

INTRODUCTION

Inadequate access to high-quality surgical services is a notable gap in the World Health Organization's (WHO) goal of improving health care delivery for all nations.[1,2] This is especially true of surgical services related to trauma, because injuries account for the greatest annual welfare lost among low and middle-income countries.[3,4] To address the deficit of surgical services, various organizations have aligned to understand and improve access to safe surgery and anesthesia to meet 80% of the world's needs by 2030.[2] The foundation of this objective lies in the coordination of multiple disciplines, including governmental organizations, nongovernmental organizations, local physicians and surgeons, and international funding sources. To achieve this 80% goal, we must first understand the global burden of surgical conditions and the resultant impact on society.[5]

Trauma to the upper extremity accounts for the majority of musculoskeletal trauma in wealthy as

Disclosure Statement: Research reported in this publication was supported by the National Institute of Arthritis and Musculoskeletal and Skin Diseases of the National Institutes of Health under Award Number 2 K24-AR053120-06. The content is solely the responsibility of the authors and does not necessarily represent the official views of the National Institutes of Health.
None of the authors has a financial interest to disclose.
Section of Plastic Surgery, Department of Surgery, University of Michigan Health System, 2130 Taubman Center, SPC 5340, 1500 East Medical Center Drive, Ann Arbor, MI 48109, USA
* Corresponding author.
E-mail address: aviram@med.umich.edu

hand.theclinics.com

well as developing nations.[4,6–10] Musculoskeletal trauma is projected to contribute 20% of the overall global burden of disease by 2020, owing largely to disability caused by these injuries.[11] Disease burden is magnified with upper extremity injuries when considering many patients who sustain these injuries are young and otherwise healthy, with much of their productivity and financial stability depending on working with their hands.[9,12–14] In developing nations, where machinery and motor vehicle injuries are more common, mutilating upper extremity trauma is a frequent cause of disability and resultant loss of productivity.[11,15,16]

Disability reflects limitations in an individual's cognitive or physical capacity that prevents completion of activities of daily living (ADLs).[17] Vulnerable populations, including those living in lower income nations, experience disability with greater prevalence than those in higher income nations.[18] As a result of a growing population of people with chronic illnesses and age-related diseases, the WHO has recently launched new programs to invest in services for the disabled and improve public awareness of these conditions.[19]

Another focus for the WHO has been on improving research strategies and quantification of data important to improving conditions among those with disabilities. The disability-adjusted life-year (DALY) is one of the most commonly used metrics to define the economic consequences and effects of morbidity and mortality on the burden of disease (**Fig. 1**). Introduced in the World Development Report in 1993, DALYs sum the total years of life lost and years of life lived with disability.[20–22] A step beyond the quality-adjusted life-year that some researchers are more familiar with, the DALY uses age weighting that helps to highlight the value of interventions that improve conditions affecting younger patients with longer time spent disabled.[23] This makes the DALY an important tool for evaluating upper extremity injuries.

By comparing the calculation of DALYs lost with and without an intervention, or between 2 interventions, it is possible to demonstrate potential economic and societal growth attributable to changes in care delivery.[20] Because the DALY quantifies

the amount of time "lost" rather than "gained" owing to a particular treatment, this metric can be used to demonstrate potential improvements foreseeable as a result of changing systems and practices currently in place. However, a major challenge in implementing these types of analyses, especially for upper extremity trauma, is how to define surgical outcomes as they relate to function and associated disability. Disability weights are notably lacking for most upper extremity conditions, especially those related to trauma.[24] Considering that upper extremity use is intricately linked to economic growth and productivity, accurately and thoughtfully measuring outcomes of upper extremity trauma treatment is critical. This is especially true for complex injuries in mutilating upper extremity trauma.

The outcomes research movement has grown as a result of an increased focus on patient-reported outcomes (PROs). As techniques for measuring and analyzing outcomes have substantially improved, the value of PROs in guiding high-quality, high-value care has been demonstrated frequently.[25,26] Although radiographs, range of motion, wound healing, or bone healing were the primary outcomes of early research, PROs, composite functional tests, and complex movement analysis are now used to provide more objective, direct measures of hand surgery outcomes. Although the value of some of these complex approaches is not yet clear, understanding the outcomes of care in terms of cost and quality has come to the forefront of research, clinical care, and health care policy around issues of resource use and distribution.

An improved understanding of outcomes has progressively changed hand and upper extremity care delivery, but these research approaches are made more difficult by the complex nature of mutilating upper extremity injuries. When considering the various mechanisms, anatomic injuries, extent of contamination, reconstruction options, and other anatomy- and injury-related variations, gathering organized and valuable data about these patients is difficult.[27] These challenges are more pronounced when evaluating mutilating upper extremity injuries across the international

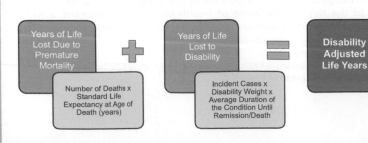

Fig. 1. Components used to calculate disability-adjusted life-years (DALY).

spectrum. Not only are there wide gaps in available resources and care infrastructure, but also different cultural and regional views on expectations and delivery of surgical care.[28–30] Despite these challenges, evaluating outcomes after surgical treatment of the mangled upper extremity is of critical importance. Unlike the lower extremity, the prosthetic options for the upper extremity remain limited and inadequate as compared with preserving a functional limb, even if not at full capacity.[31,32] Salvage treatment for patients with mutilating upper extremity injuries remains a top priority so that outcomes can be optimized and patients can return to function and gainful employment as often as possible. Measuring and understanding outcomes after mutilating upper extremity injuries is critical for improving care and quality of life for these injured patients.

In this article, we review techniques used for measuring outcomes after upper extremity surgery, the challenges associated with using these techniques for the patient with a mutilating hand injury, and the potential value of these instruments for patients of varying demographics and regions across the globe.

MEASURING OUTCOMES

With the increased focus on understanding outcomes has come a wave of new measurement approaches and tools. Certainly, understanding how a patient is able to move and function after an upper extremity injury is important. However, as we engage in understanding the multidimensional facets of functional recovery on a patient's psychosocial well-being and their interaction with the external environment, such as their family, their work place, and society, a holistic concept of health-related quality of life (HRQL) has developed.[23,33] Quality of life is an interactive tenet with contributing influence from psychological, physical, functional, and social factors. Additionally, related economic and spiritual/religious elements can have an effect. HRQL describes how these components of a patient's life are affected by their health condition and health status.[17,34–36]

The movement to understand HRQL and related elements of posttraumatic recovery has drawn attention to understanding PROs. By allowing patients to report on their condition and ability to function, we have gained insights into overall disability beyond simple anatomic evaluations or basic functional tests. These approaches have shown the importance of understanding returning to function and work, mental health and coping, and other critical components of postinjury support that contribute to long-term treatment success.

One of the critical elements to understanding outcomes after upper extremity trauma is the distinction between impairment and disability. Impairment is defined as "an alteration of an individual's health status – a deviation from normal in a body part or organ system and its functioning," whereas disability is defined as "an alteration of an individual's capacity to meet personal, social, or occupational demands because of an impairment."[37,38] For some patients they are related, but in many cases, a patient's anatomic impairment does not correlate to their degree of disability.[39,40] Some patients with less severe injuries are functionally limited, yet others with mutilating injuries find ways to return to useful function, even with severe impairment.[41] This gap is often accentuated when evaluating patients with external pressures to optimize function.

MEASUREMENT APPROACHES AND TECHNIQUES

Although PROs are immensely valuable in measuring posttraumatic outcomes, applying standardized norms and comparing scores across PROs defined in high-income countries may result in inaccurate comparisons in measured impairment and disability among patients in developing nations. Many of these patients are potentially more likely to overcome obstacles to return to adequate function so they can provide for themselves and their families. Although these external pressures may result in an optimization of outcomes, they also make understanding treatment outcomes as well as the gap between impairment and disability an even greater challenge. For some patients, using a traditional strength, range of motion, and composite functional tests, especially as they relate to PROs, may be of great value in helping understand which treatments are better than others. The complex and variable nature of the injuries necessitates a comprehensive multimodal approach to measuring outcomes after mutilating upper extremity trauma.

Functional Testing

Traditionally, outcomes studies are centered on strength, range of motion, and sensory tests. For strength testing, grip, 3-finger pinch, key pinch, and many others have been used routinely, with technique descriptions and standardized instruments available.[42] However, even if these tools are not available to investigators with limited resources, these strength metrics can be tested other ways as long as the methods are reproducible and standardized across patients and measurement episodes.[43]

For sensory testing, Semmes-Weinstein monofilaments and 2-point discrimination are used frequently, although many others exist.[44,45] These techniques can evaluate static and dynamic sensory function, vibratory and pressure sensation, and sensory acuity. Although the technique used across testers is somewhat more susceptible to variation and inconsistency than the strength tests, these sensory metrics all have standard techniques for use that can be taught.[46]

The appeal of these tests is that they are easy to perform, reproducible, understood by patients and providers, and can be compared among studies. As a result, many of them have become commonplace in the discussion of treatment outcomes after upper extremity surgery. However, they do not provide a complete understanding of function. As a result, composite functional testing is also used frequently.

Composite functional tests aim to evaluate the patient's use of the entire limb, and often test fine and gross motor tasks. Some also include tests that evaluate composite ADLs as a way to evaluate a patient's ability to function independently with their condition. Each method differs in approach to testing function and ADLs, with varying clinimetric properties and overall utility in understanding the condition of the upper limb.[47,48] One shortcoming of these tests is that they often use time as a gauge for success and adequate performance, which introduces additional biases and inaccuracies in measurement unrelated to isolated limb recovery and function (eg, visual acuity, baseline tremors, traumatic head injuries, and others). Age-based normative values have been reported for some tests, helping to reduce that measurement inaccuracy over groups of patients.[49–52]

More recently, biomechanics and kinesiology specialists have worked to devise technology-based approaches to testing strength, range of motion, and function of the upper limb.[53–55] Across these composite and biomechanical tests, none has been shown repeatedly to be better than the others; however, most provide some useful information. Additionally, similar to the static tests described, these approaches provide a standardized and reproducible way to evaluate function.

Many consider these functional tests, especially the digitized strength and range of motion measurement tools, to be more "objective" measures; however, the amount of effort and force a patient puts in to the test, as well as reporting accurately for sensory testing, can all be altered by the patient if they choose to do so.[56,57] Therefore, the terms objective and subjective should be eliminated in any hand functional measures because the patient, based on their effort and intangible motivation, can influence them all. Where these tests are notably lacking is in the ability to measure and report on psychosocial aspects of recovery that are not directly related to function. As a result, researchers and providers use PROs to fill those knowledge gaps.

Patient-Reported Outcomes Measurements

The patient-centered outcomes movement has increasingly put value on reporting, understanding, and optimizing HRQL. Understanding how to consistently improve HRQL after treating a condition, while minimizing excess spending and waste, is important to providers, economists, health systems, patients, and society as a whole.[26,58] In efforts toward reaching this goal, the value and importance of PROs has grown immensely. It has been demonstrated repeatedly that allowing patients to report on their conditions provides unique and reliable insight into their recovery and overall condition.

PROs are obtained through questionnaires. The questionnaires focus on general, system-specific, or condition-specific HRQL.[26] Many measures evaluate how patients believe they are able to perform critical ADLs. To be used for research and outcomes measurements, these questionnaires are thoroughly evaluated for numerous metrics, including reliability, validity, and reproducibility (**Table 1**). Questionnaire results can then be compared across studies and among conditions. Critics regard these PROs as subjective and potentially manipulated by patients with ulterior motives; however, they are no more easily manipulated than the functional tests, and in many cases provide unique insights that the functional tests cannot evaluate.

Challenges in the Mangled Extremity Patient

PROs after upper extremity trauma, when followed over time, often show improvement in HRQL.[59] Some of this is attributable to recovery but some is also related to patients adjusting to their conditions.[30] The ability to adjust to a condition varies. Patients from different financial, cultural, and regional backgrounds may approach their treatment, rehabilitation, and outcomes differently.[60] Considering that a substantial volume of these injuries occur among patients in developing nations, we must think about the different experiences these patients have in dealing with upper extremity trauma compared with those in higher income nations. The absence of adequate social services, rehabilitation, and financial support for families creates a different series of motivations for these patients to push through their recovery.[61] Additionally, these differences will change how patients

Table 1
Definitions for key measurement properties used in evaluating the quality of patient-reported outcomes instruments

Measurement Property	Definition
Content validity	Degree to which the content of an instrument is an adequate reflection of the construct being measured
Criterion validity	Strength of relationship between questionnaire scores and a measurable criterion ("gold standard")
Construct validity	Degree to which the scores of a questionnaire are consistent with the theoretic construct (hypothesis) being measured
Face validity	Degree to which items in an instrument look as though they are an adequate reflection of the construct being measured
Internal consistency	Extent to which the items are interrelated, and thus measure the same construct
Reliability	Extent to which patients can be distinguished from each other despite measurement errors
Test–retest reliability	Extent to which scores for patients who have not changed are the same in repeated measurements over time
Interrater reliability	Extent to which scores for patients who have not changed are the same over repeated measurements by different examiners during the same visit
Responsiveness	Ability to detect clinically meaningful change over time in the construct being measured
Interpretability	Degree to which quantitative scores can be given qualitative meaning. Identifying clinically important differences in results.
Cross-cultural equivalence	The same measurement instrument used in different cultures measures the same construct without additional external cultural influences on results

report their outcomes, increasing the difficulty with which these treatments and results can be studied in a systematic fashion. Most of what we know about PROs has come from patients and studies in wealthy nations. Interpreting and translating PRO results from patients in the developing world is likely different from patients in wealthy nations, and may limit how well these metrics reflect long-term functional outcomes and disability.

Improvements in data collection and databases provide new ways to analyze group data to evaluate systems of care and use.[62] Whether using patient databases for clinical trial and outcomes studies, or larger state or national databases for "big data" studies, improvements in data collection and organization have opened doors to answering many new and challenging questions. Additionally, by pooling data, researchers are able to evaluate components of care that otherwise could not be properly analyzed owing to smaller patient numbers or too little variation in small outcomes studies. However, larger database approaches are a challenge for evaluating the treatment of mutilating upper extremity injuries because of variability inherent in these traumas.

This is made more difficult by the variations in treatment approaches and options for these patients. This heterogeneity results in limited usefulness of the currently available large databases for studying these types of injuries, and makes it difficult to organize a clinical study evaluating mutilating hand injury treatments and outcomes with most of the resources available today. Additionally, much of the available data in trauma registries has inconsistent quality, especially for data from developing nations.[27]

Another challenge in using PROs to evaluate massive upper extremity trauma is that these questionnaires are mostly all written in English and geared toward Western society with certain values and norms.[63] As a result, using these PROs globally requires accurate translation (**Fig. 2**) and cross-cultural validation.[64] This is especially important when attempting to gain insights into elements such as satisfaction that can largely depend on expectations and goals.[63,65] Patients in developing nations may have different approaches to their care, and that may be reflected in how they consider and respond to items in questionnaires. This may also limit the comparability of PRO results

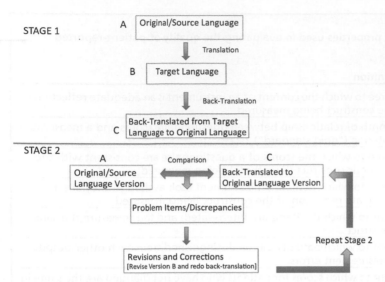

Fig. 2. Flow diagram for the process of translating a patient-reported outcomes questionnaire. (*Adapted from* Sperber AD. Translation and validation of study instruments for cross-cultural research. Gastroenterology 2004;126(1 Suppl 1):S126; with permission.)

from different patient populations in ways unique to international research. As researchers look to use these translated instruments in the international arena, it will be important to validate them across the different cultures and populations of interest, including comparisons to some of the functional metrics, similar to what has been done in English-speaking countries.

VALIDATION OF PATIENT-REPORTED OUTCOMES

A key step is to validate PROs for use in this population. As described, there are metrics used to evaluate the questionnaires, and confirming that these questionnaires correlate to the traditional measures of recovery—strength, sensation, composite function, and so on—is an essential step in that process. This has already been done for some questionnaires and, although the sample populations for the validations studies are somewhat limited, these questionnaires should be used in future studies. Most notably, the Michigan Hand Questionnaire[66,67] and the Disability of the Arm, Shoulder, and Hand questionnaire[68] have been used frequently and evaluated with the upper extremity trauma patient.[69,70] With the addition of an aesthetic element and greater focus on satisfaction and HRQL, the Michigan Hand Questionnaire often correlates more strongly with mental health outcomes than other upper extremity questionnaires.[39] Although the impact of this finding is not yet clear, especially as it relates to measuring quality of overall care and long-term disability, it illustrates how across validated PROs there can still be variations in the findings. Understanding the

different benefits and downsides of the questionnaires helps in choosing the appropriate metric to use for each research question.[71,72] It is also important to consider the factors that can affect questionnaire responses (**Box 1**) and mitigate

---

Box 1
Factors affecting accurate completion of questionnaires

Patient Factors

Literacy

Comprehension

Mental and emotional state

Personality

Fatigue

Secondary gain

Questionnaire Factors

Length

Clarity

Applicability and relevance of content

Other

Environment

Compensation

Ongoing litigation

Family or caregiver influence

Adapted from Bindra RR, Dias JJ, Heras-Palau C, et al. Assessing outcome after hand surgery: the current state. J Hand Surg Br 2003;28(4):291; with permission.

them as best as possible in designing and implementing a study.[73]

One study that aimed at answering the question of how the functional measures relate to the PROs, and how both of these outcomes contribute to overall functional disability, highlights the complex interplay between these elements. In this study, finger amputation patients performed functional tests and completed PRO questionnaires.[39] They also had anatomic injury ("impairment") measured based on a standardized weighting system by digit and length lost. The patients then performed complex functional tasks as a measure of their ability to perform ADLs and as a way to reflect overall disability. In this study, the upper extremity PROs not only correlated with the functional tests, but they also correlated with mental health and HRQL questionnaires, and overall composite function and disability. The impairment score, reflecting anatomic injury, did not correlate with performance and overall disability. This study confirms the importance of measuring outcomes after upper extremity injuries and of using instruments that will reflect total composite function and not just see the anatomic injury as the only element in recovery.

Where this becomes even more important is in translating PROs and the results of these studies to the developing world. In these patients, the degree of anatomic injury is potentially less likely to predict outcomes and return to function. The external motivation to optimize recovery is different in those cultures and economic systems. As a result, aspects of rehabilitation care systems, returning to work, and patient participation also must be evaluated to understand the recovery process fully. Considering the impact that a return to function can have for these patients, it is even more important that we find ways to measure outcomes and improve care in the resource-limited setting.

APPLICATIONS IN RESEARCH

The available literature on outcomes after mutilating upper extremity trauma is sparse. Although a few larger case series as well as large database studies exist, the vast majority are published using small case series and single-surgeon or single-center experiences that focus on distal amputations and replantation. Within high-income nations, documenting the consequences of severe mangling and proximal injuries is limited to small series as a result of the low incidence of these injuries. In developing nations where these injuries are more common, the lack of access to proper surgical services and research support limits the opportunity to gain perspective on these injuries regardless of the high incidence.

However, we have developed great knowledge from what is presented in the upper extremity trauma outcomes literature. By measuring outcomes after surgical treatment of the traumatized upper extremity, we have an improved understanding of external fixation versus internal fixation techniques, methods to optimize bone healing, timing of reconstruction, replantation techniques, and much more. Notably, the value of replantation and complex salvage of the mangled upper extremity has been evaluated.[74–76] The early outcomes research for these injuries has paved the way for the complex care and complex research methodology.

As we look to improve how we measure outcomes in these patients, the focus has shifted to improving use of PROs to understand the complexities of recovery, functionality, and associated disability from these injuries. Through this information not only can we guide appropriate care to improve outcomes, but also establish the value of upper extremity salvage, the need for services in resource-limited settings, and approaches to optimize care of the upper extremity trauma patient. Additionally, as treatment guidelines and care criteria are established, data collection can be done in a more organized and systematic way to build databases and facilitate larger studies.

One of the next steps is to develop a core outcomes set to be used for all upper extremity trauma studies.[77] This set should be based on a conceptual framework of health, and vetted thoroughly to determine the best set of outcome measures to encompass all critical elements of recovery after upper extremity trauma. This will help to minimize confusion across studies, facilitate better cross-study comparisons, and reduce inconsistencies in data collection and reporting to begin addressing the gaps in available data and measured outcomes after upper extremity reconstruction and salvage.

IMPACT AND RELATED RESEARCH

Beyond measuring outcomes, there are related areas of research that help clarify the impact of understanding how these patients recover after injury. To evaluate the true economic implications of mutilating hand injuries in developing nations, we must first identify the percentage of musculoskeletal trauma that is related to upper extremity injury, and to define the incidence and prevalence of this particular trauma. Although studies have been performed to evaluate the global burden of surgically treatable conditions as a whole, additional studies are required to understand the epidemiology, mechanisms of injury, and environmental exposures that contribute to the globally high incidence of trauma in a condition-specific manner.[18,24,78] Given the basic principle that the economic and societal burden of surgical disease is based on the incidence and prevalence of any condition, global estimates of upper extremity trauma are critical—not only to understand the need for care delivery, but also to add value to improvements we can make in treatment outcomes and optimization.[5]

We must create an accurate metric of disability among patients with hand injuries to improve the generalizability of findings as we move forward with additional studies. This approach ties in closely with the concept of creating a core set of outcomes measures to use in all upper extremity trauma studies. The inextricable link between hand injuries, functional outcomes, and occupational consequences is likely underestimated and underreported in the absence of such a system. Although the DALY is a useful measure that can be compared across conditions and populations, some have suggested that categorizing surgical needs into met, unmet, and unmeetable needs is a more practical method. Calculating "effective coverage," as a metric of met need compared with overall need, would promote countries to more effectively plan and improve access to care for conditions that place the greatest burden on society.[79] Different nations have different needs, and the benefits of adding and expanding surgical services vary based on the unmet needs in different regions. Understanding these variations across the international spectrum will guide prioritizing care delivery.

Another novel approach to evaluating the disability burden owing to a condition is the Model Disability Survey, piloted by the WHO and the World Bank.[80] The Model Disability Survey avoids using surveyors who often underreport patients with mild to moderate disability, and instead compares affected with nonaffected patients to determine disability criteria. Such improved evaluation and capture of disabled persons is a substantial step toward understanding injury burden, and could benefit the study of upper extremity disability after trauma. This, alongside improvements in understanding what treatments and approaches optimize outcomes, will facilitate improvement in the care of these patients worldwide.

One of the most important elements is to establish that high-quality outcomes can be obtained in the resource-limited setting. This has been done by the Ganga hospital group, along with select others.[16,74] Complex reconstruction can be performed in these settings. Until recently, the need in these regions has largely been ignored aside from intermittent mission work. Mission trips focused on hand surgery are thought to be cost effective in that the cost per DALY averted is less than twice the per capita gross national income.[81] Although mission trips are important to minimize the continued disability associated with remote injuries, it is only by having well-trained local providers that a sustainable system is achieved.[82] This includes availability of complex reconstruction and microsurgery. Current data reflect an overall limited number of orthopedic and plastic surgeons practicing in the developing world, where need for these services is high.[83] For example, in the United States and Canada there is 1 plastic surgeon per 57,000 people. In India and China, there are 1.5 plastic surgeons for every 1 million people. In sub-Saharan Africa, there are even fewer providers—Ghana has 6 plastic surgeons for 22 million people and Uganda has 3 plastic surgeons for 27 million people.[83,84] As we improve our understanding of treatment outcomes, disseminating this information to frontline providers will aid in optimizing quality and triage of the limited care that can be delivered by the available surgeons.

The cost effectiveness of surgical interventions overall compares favorably to that of vaccines. Although the cost of vaccinations is $5 for every DALY averted, the cost of surgery is slightly higher at $11 to 77 per DALY averted.[85] In developing nations, the cost is on the lower end of that range because the DALY benefit for the same procedures is often higher.[86] Improving care and associated outcomes will only make reconstructive upper extremity surgery more valuable. Given the importance of hand function on all aspects of economic productivity, as plastic and orthopedic surgeons we must clearly delineate the contributions of hand injuries to this system. By defining the proper metrics, disease-specific factors, and modeling schematics unique to treating mutilating hand injuries, we can create an environment of sustainable progress within middle- and low-income nations.

SUMMARY

Measuring outcomes after massive upper extremity trauma is a critical yet difficult task, made more complicated by the various cultures and regions affected by these types of traumatic events. As a result, a comprehensive approach to this international problem is warranted, one that combines the various modalities in a way that promotes thorough outcomes measurement, consistent and reliable reporting, and an ability to improve our understanding of treatment quality and value as they relate to long-term disability and patient satisfaction. As this information becomes available, it must be spread to the already overburdened providers in the developing world, so that they may optimize care systems and care delivery for this high-need population. This has unique implications for the developing world, where economics of care place even greater value on capacity building, quality improvement, and high-yield approaches to complex surgical challenges.

REFERENCES

1. Farmer PE, Kim JY. Surgery and global health: a view from beyond the OR. World J Surg 2008;32(4):533–6.
2. Meara JG, Leather AJ, Hagander L, et al. Global Surgery 2030: evidence and solutions for achieving health, welfare, and economic development. Int J Obstet Anesth 2016;25:75–8.
3. Alkire BC, Shrime MG, Dare AJ, et al. Global economic consequences of selected surgical diseases: a modelling study. Lancet Glob Health 2015;3(Suppl 2):S21–7.
4. Alkire BC, Vincent JR, Meara JG. Benefit-cost analysis for selected surgical interventions in low- and middle-income countries. In: Debas HT, Donkor P, Gawande A, et al, editors. Essential surgery: disease control priorities. 3rd edition. vol. 1. Washington, DC: World Bank; 2015.
5. Rose J, Weiser TG, Hider P, et al. Estimated need for surgery worldwide based on prevalence of diseases: a modelling strategy for the WHO Global Health Estimate. Lancet Glob Health 2015;3(Suppl 2):S13–20.
6. Linden AF, Maine R, Hedt-Gauthier BL, et al. Epidemiology of untreated non-obstetric surgical disease in Burera District, Rwanda: a Cross-sectional Survey. Lancet 2015;385(Suppl 2):S9.
7. Brouillette MA, Kaiser SP, Konadu P, et al. Orthopedic surgery in the developing world: workforce and operative volumes in Ghana compared to those in the United States. World J Surg 2014;38(4):849–57.
8. Mehrpour SR, Nabian MH, Oryadi Zanjani L, et al. Descriptive epidemiology of traumatic injuries in 18890 adults: a 5-year-study in a tertiary trauma center in Iran. Asian J Sports Med 2015;6(1): e23129.
9. Gaul JS Jr. Identifiable costs and tangible benefits resulting from the treatment of acute injuries of the hand. J Hand Surg 1987;12(5 Pt 2):966–70.
10. McCall BP, Horwitz IB. An assessment and quantification of the rates, costs, and risk factors of occupational amputations: analysis of Kentucky workers' compensation claims, 1994-2003. Am J Ind Med 2006;49(12):1031–8.
11. Beveridge M, Howard A. The burden of orthopaedic disease in developing countries. J Bone Joint Surg Am 2004;86-A(8):1819–22.
12. Dias JJ, Garcia-Elias M. Hand injury costs. Injury Nov 2006;37(11):1071–7.
13. Holmberg J, Lindgren B, Jutemark R. Replantation-revascularization and primary amputation in major hand injuries. Resources spent on treatment and the indirect costs of sick leave in Sweden. J Hand Surg 1996;21(5):576–80.
14. de Putter CE, Selles RW, Polinder S, et al. Economic impact of hand and wrist injuries: health-care costs and productivity costs in a population-based study. J Bone Joint Surg Am 2012;94(9):e56.
15. Omoke NI, Chukwu CO, Madubueze CC, et al. Traumatic extremity amputation in a Nigerian setting: patterns and challenges of care. Int Orthop 2012;36(3):613–8.
16. Sabapathy SR, Satbhai NG. Microsurgery in the urgent and emergent management of the hand. Curr Rev Musculoskelet Med 2014;7(1):40–6.
17. Verbrugge LM, Jette AM. The disablement process. Soc Sci Med 1994;38(1):1–14.
18. World report on Disability 2011. Geneva: World Bank and WHO; 2011.
19. MacLachlan M, Mannan H. The World Report on Disability and its implications for rehabilitation psychology. Rehabil Psychol 2014;59(2):117–24.
20. Fox-Rushby JA, Hanson K. Calculating and presenting disability adjusted life years (DALYs) in cost-effectiveness analysis. Health Policy Plan 2001; 16(3):326–31.
21. Musgrove P. Investing in health: the 1993 World Development Report of the World Bank. Bull Pan Am Health Organ 1993;27(3):284–6.
22. Murray CJ. Quantifying the burden of disease: the technical basis for disability-adjusted life years. Bull World Health Organ 1994;72(3):429–45.
23. Sassi F. Calculating QALYs, comparing QALY and DALY calculations. Health Policy Plan 2006;21(5): 402–8.
24. GBD 2013 DALYs and HALE Collaborators, Murray CJ, Barber RM, et al. Global, regional, and national disability-adjusted life years (DALYs) for 306 diseases and injuries and healthy life expectancy (HALE) for 188 countries, 1990-2013: quantifying the epidemiological transition. Lancet 2015; 386(10009):2145–91.
25. Alderman AK, Chung KC. Measuring outcomes in hand surgery. Clin Plast Surg 2008;35(2):239–50.
26. Giladi AM, Chung KC. Measuring outcomes in hand surgery. Clin Plast Surg 2013;40(2):313–22.
27. O'Reilly GM, Gabbe B, Moore L, et al. Classifying, measuring and improving the quality of data in trauma registries: a review of the literature. Injury 2016;47(3):559–67.
28. Breslau J. Cultures of trauma: anthropological views of posttraumatic stress disorder in international

health. Cult Med Psychiatry 2004;28(2):113–26 [discussion: 211–20].

29. Wee JY. Adjusting expectations after spinal cord injury across global settings: a commentary. Disabil Rehabil 2006;28(10):659–61.

30. Chan J, Spencer J. Adaptation to hand injury: an evolving experience. Am J Occup Ther 2004;58(2):128–39.

31. Graham B, Adkins P, Tsai TM, et al. Major replantation versus revision amputation and prosthetic fitting in the upper extremity: a late functional outcomes study. J Hand Surg 1998;23(5):783–91.

32. Stanger K, Horch RE, Dragu A. Severe mutilating injuries with complex macroamputations of the upper extremity - is it worth the effort? World J Emerg Surg 2015;10:30.

33. Guyatt GH, Feeny DH, Patrick DL. Measuring health-related quality of life. Ann Intern Med 1993;118(8):622–9.

34. Barbier O, Penta M, Thonnard JL. Outcome evaluation of the hand and wrist according to the International Classification of Functioning, Disability, and Health. Hand Clin 2003;19(3):371–8, vii.

35. Gill TM, Feinstein AR. A critical appraisal of the quality of quality-of-life measurements. JAMA 1994;272(8):619–26.

36. Garratt A, Schmidt L, Mackintosh A, et al. Quality of life measurement: bibliographic study of patient assessed health outcome measures. BMJ 2002;324(7351):1417.

37. Rondinelli RE. Guides to the evaluation of permanent impairment. 6th edition. Chicago (IL): American Medical Association; 2008.

38. Wood PH. Appreciating the consequences of disease: the international classification of impairments, disabilities, and handicaps. WHO Chron 1980;34(10):376–80.

39. Giladi AM, McGlinn EP, Shauver MJ, et al. Measuring outcomes and determining long-term disability after revision amputation for treatment of traumatic finger and thumb amputation injuries. Plast Reconstr Surg 2014;134(5):746e–55e.

40. van Oosterom FJ, Ettema AM, Mulder PG, et al. Impairment and disability after severe hand injuries with multiple phalangeal fractures. J Hand Surg 2007;32(1):91–5.

41. Lee YY, Chang JH, Shieh SJ, et al. Association between the initial anatomical severity and opportunity of return to work in occupational hand injured patients. J Trauma 2010;69(6):E88–93.

42. Mathiowetz V, Kashman N, Volland G, et al. Grip and pinch strength: normative data for adults. Arch Phys Med Rehabil 1985;66(2):69–74.

43. Wells R, Greig M. Characterizing human hand prehensile strength by force and moment wrench. Ergonomics 2001;44(15):1392–402.

44. Moberg E. Two-point discrimination test. A valuable part of hand surgical rehabilitation, e.g. in tetraplegia. Scand J Rehabil Med 1990;22(3):127–34.

45. Bell-Krotoski J. Advances in sensibility evaluation. Hand Clin 1991;7(3):527–46.

46. Lehman LF, Orsini MB, Nicholl AR. The development and adaptation of the Semmes-Weinstein monofilaments in Brazil. J Hand Ther 1993;6(4):290–7.

47. van de Ven-Stevens LA, Munneke M, Terwee CB, et al. Clinimetric properties of instruments to assess activities in patients with hand injury: a systematic review of the literature. Arch Phys Med Rehabil 2009;90(1):151–69.

48. Schoneveld K, Wittink H, Takken T. Clinimetric evaluation of measurement tools used in hand therapy to assess activity and participation. J Hand Ther 2009;22(3):221–35 [quiz: 236].

49. Van Harlinger W, Blalock L, Merritt JL. Upper limb strength: study providing normative data for a clinical handheld dynamometer. PM R 2015;7(2):135–40.

50. McQuiddy VA, Scheerer CR, Lavalley R, et al. Normative Values for grip and pinch strength for 6- to 19-Year-Olds. Arch Phys Med Rehabil 2015;96(9):1627–33.

51. Desrosiers J, Hebert R, Bravo G, et al. The Purdue Pegboard Test: normative data for people aged 60 and over. Disabil Rehabil 1995;17(5):217–24.

52. Amirjani N, Ashworth NL, Gordon T, et al. Normative values and the effects of age, gender, and handedness on the Moberg Pick-Up Test. Muscle Nerve 2007;35(6):788–92.

53. van Huizum MA, Hoornweg MJ, de Ruiter N, et al. Effect of latissimus dorsi flap breast reconstruction on the strength profile of the upper extremity. J Plast Surg Hand Surg 2016;50(4):202–7.

54. Holzbaur KR, Murray WM, Delp SL. A model of the upper extremity for simulating musculoskeletal surgery and analyzing neuromuscular control. Ann Biomed Eng 2005;33(6):829–40.

55. Cui PH, Visell Y. Linear and nonlinear subspace analysis of hand movements during grasping. Conf Proc IEEE Eng Med Biol Soc 2014;2014:2529–32.

56. Robinson ME, Dannecker EA. Critical issues in the use of muscle testing for the determination of sincerity of effort. Clin J Pain 2004;20(6):392–8.

57. Fairfax AH, Balnave R, Adams RD. Variability of grip strength during isometric contraction. Ergonomics 1995;38(9):1819–30.

58. Wilson IB, Cleary PD. Linking clinical variables with health-related quality of life. A conceptual model of patient outcomes. JAMA 1995;273(1):59–65.

59. Kovacs L, Grob M, Zimmermann A, et al. Quality of life after severe hand injury. J Plast Reconstr Aesthet Surg 2011;64(11):1495–502.

60. Myers NL. Culture stress and recovery from schizophrenia: lessons from the field for global mental health. Cult Med Psychiatry 2010;34(3):500–28.

61. Harris I, Mulford J, Solomon M, et al. Association between compensation status and outcome after surgery: a meta-analysis. JAMA 2005;293(13):1644–52.

62. Malay S, Shauver MJ, Chung KC. Applicability of large databases in outcomes research. J Hand Surg 2012;37(7):1437–46.

63. Gonzalez-Calvo J, Gonzalez VM, Lorig K. Cultural diversity issues in the development of valid and reliable measures of health status. Arthritis Care Res 1997;10(6):448–56.

64. Sperber AD. Translation and validation of study instruments for cross-cultural research. Gastroenterology 2004;126(1 Suppl 1):S124–8.

65. Van Ommeren M. Validity issues in transcultural epidemiology. Br J Psychiatry 2003;182:376–8.

66. Chung KC, Pillsbury MS, Walters MR, et al. Reliability and validity testing of the Michigan Hand Outcomes Questionnaire. J Hand Surg 1998;23(4):575–87.

67. Chung KC, Hamill JB, Walters MR, et al. The Michigan Hand Outcomes Questionnaire (MHQ): assessment of responsiveness to clinical change. Ann Plast Surg 1999;42(6):619–22.

68. Hudak PL, Amadio PC, Bombardier C. Development of an upper extremity outcome measure: the DASH (disabilities of the arm, shoulder and hand) [corrected]. The Upper Extremity Collaborative Group (UECG). Am J Ind Med 1996;29(6):602–8.

69. Voineskos SH, Coroneos CJ, Thoma A, et al. Measuring and understanding treatment effectiveness in hand surgery. Hand Clin 2014;30(3):285–92, v.

70. Hoang-Kim A, Pegreffi F, Moroni A, et al. Measuring wrist and hand function: common scales and checklists. Injury 2011;42(3):253–8.

71. Changulani M, Okonkwo U, Keswani T, et al. Outcome evaluation measures for wrist and hand: which one to choose? Int Orthop 2008;32(1):1–6.

72. Sears ED, Chung KC. A guide to interpreting a study of patient-reported outcomes. Plast Reconstr Surg 2012;129(5):1200–7.

73. Bindra RR, Dias JJ, Heras-Palau C, et al. Assessing outcome after hand surgery: the current state. J Hand Surg 2003;28(4):289–94.

74. Sabapathy SR, Venkatramani H, Bharathi RR, et al. Technical considerations and functional outcome of 22 major replantations (The BSSH Douglas Lamb Lecture, 2005). J Hand Surg Eur 2007;32(5):488–501.

75. Chuang DC, Lai JB, Cheng SL, et al. Traction avulsion amputation of the major upper limb: a proposed new classification, guidelines for acute management, and strategies for secondary reconstruction. Plast Reconstr Surg 2001;108(6):1624–38.

76. Manord JD, Garrard CL, Kline DG, et al. Management of severe proximal vascular and neural injury of the upper extremity. J Vasc Surg 1998;27(1):43–7 [discussion: 48–9].

77. Idzerda L, Rader T, Tugwell P, et al. Can we decide which outcomes should be measured in every clinical trial? A scoping review of the existing conceptual frameworks and processes to develop core outcome sets. J Rheumatol 2014;41(5):986–93.

78. Poenaru D. The burden of pediatric surgical disease in low-resource settings: Discovering it, measuring it, and addressing it. J Pediatr Surg 2016;51(2):216–20.

79. Poenaru D, Ozgediz D, Gosselin RA. Burden, need, or backlog: a call for improved metrics for the global burden of surgical disease. Int J Surg 2014;12(5):483–6.

80. Sabariego C, Oberhauser C, Posarac A, et al. Measuring disability: comparing the impact of two data collection approaches on disability rates. Int J Environ Res Public Health 2015;12(9):10329–51.

81. Tadisina KK, Chopra K, Tangredi J, et al. Helping hands: a cost-effectiveness study of a humanitarian hand surgery mission. Plast Surg Int 2014;2014:921625.

82. Shrime MG, Sleemi A, Ravilla TD. Charitable platforms in global surgery: a systematic review of their effectiveness, cost-effectiveness, sustainability, and role training. World J Surg 2015;39(1):10–20.

83. Semer NB, Sullivan SR, Meara JG. Plastic surgery and global health: how plastic surgery impacts the global burden of surgical disease. J Plast Reconstr Aesthet Surg 2010;63(8):1244–8.

84. Gosselin RA, Thind A, Bellardinelli A. Cost/DALY averted in a small hospital in Sierra Leone: what is the relative contribution of different services? World J Surg 2006;30(4):505–11.

85. Mock CN, Donkor P, Gawande A, et al. Essential surgery: key messages of this volume. In: Debas HT, Donkor P, Gawande A, et al, editors. Essential surgery: disease control priorities. 3rd edition. vol. 1. Washington, DC: World Bank; 2015.

86. Poenaru D, Pemberton J, Frankfurter C, et al. Quantifying the disability from congenital anomalies averted through pediatric surgery: a cross-sectional comparison of a pediatric surgical unit in Kenya and Canada. World J Surg 2015;39(9):2198–206.

Mutilating Hand Injuries in Children

Sunil M. Thirkannad, MD

KEYWORDS

- Hand injury • Child • Mutilating • Replantation • Revascularization • Trauma • Burns

KEY POINTS

- Mutilating hand injuries in children are significant because of the actual tissue injury and the significant psychological impact they have on the patient and family.
- Management of these injuries requires significant surgical skill as well as a well-planned and well-executed treatment protocol.
- This article discusses the etiology, incidence, and treatment of mutilating hand injuries in a child.
- The relevant literature has been reviewed and appropriate treatment guidelines have been provided.

INTRODUCTION

Children are naturally curious! Anything and everything within hand's reach will be probed. This renders the upper extremity and particularly the hand vulnerable to injury. In addition, it is but natural for a human being to thrust out one's hands as a means of protection from a fall or as a means of shielding oneself from approaching danger. This in turn further increases the risk of injury.[1]

EPIDEMIOLOGY

An exhaustive analysis of injuries in children between the ages of 0 and 19 years was conducted by the Centers for Disease Control and Prevention, evaluating data between 2001 and 2006.[2] This revealed an average of 11,272 nonfatal injuries per 100,000 population with a majority of them occurring in males (58%). An interesting finding of the study was that these injuries demonstrated 2 peaks in age incidence. The first peak was between 1 and 4 years of age and the second between 15 and 19 years of age–with the lowest incidence being in children under the age of 1 year. This apparently skewed incidence of nonfatal injuries in children seems to follow characteristic phases in the interaction of a developing child with the external environment. A child between the ages of 1 and 4 years is just making his or her first foray into the new world. It is this child who is most inquisitive and hence most likely to probe and investigate every unfamiliar object and thus get injured. In a similar manner, children between the ages of 15 and 19 years are typically leaving the protected confines of their homes for the first time and venturing out on their own. These behavior patterns render children more vulnerable to injuries and are further exemplified by the type of injury sustained. Fortunately, there has been a slow but steady decrease in the incidence of nonfatal injuries over time. Studies have revealed that a total of 14,475 nonfatal injuries were reported in 2000 and that number decreased to 11,392 in 2013, a total decrease of 22% over a 13-year period.[3]

Our institution has seen a steady decrease in the number of mutilating injuries seen in children over the years. Between 1970 and 1979, we performed 60 replants in 41 children.[4] A subsequent study looked at data over a 15-year period from 1973 to 1988 and found that a total of 62 pediatric

Disclosure: The author has not received nor will receive any financial consideration for part or whole of this study.
Christine M. Kleinert Institute for Hand & Microsurgery, KleinertKutz Hand Care Center, University of Louisville, 225 Abraham Flexner Way, Suite 810, Louisville, KY 40202, USA
E-mail address: sthirkannad@kleinertkutz.com

Hand Clin 32 (2016) 477–489
http://dx.doi.org/10.1016/j.hcl.2016.07.007
0749-0712/16/© 2016 Elsevier Inc. All rights reserved.

amputations were seen in our practice but only 32 digits in 29 patients were found replantable.[5] Over the last decade, replantations and revascularizations in children have dwindled to single digits each year in our institution, although the adult numbers have remained constant at around a 100 patients. This fortunate decrease in the incidence of severe mutilating injuries in children can be attributed to significant improvements in safety features in toys, furniture, and other household goods, compounded by an increase in awareness among the general public.

ETIOLOGY

Mutilating hand injuries in children are as a result of direct trauma to the hand. Broadly, these injuries can be placed under 3 categories: accidental, nonaccidental (abuse) and self-mutilation. Accidental injuries are by far the commonest cause of injury and in turn may be divided into those caused by direct trauma and those owing to burns. Explosions, which by nature can cause devastating injuries, present with a combination of injury patterns and have elements of both direct trauma and burns. The report from the Centers for Disease Control an Prevention on injuries in children found that overall, falls were the commonest reason for injuries in children between the ages of 1 and 4 years; in contrast, being struck by an object was the commonest reason for injury in children between 15 and 19 years.[2] However, mutilating hand injuries in our experience have shown a slightly different pattern of causation compared with the general pattern of upper extremity injuries. In younger children, the commonest reason for amputation of a digit has been a crush injury, with the hand most often caught in something that shuts (door, window, car door, lid of a heavy box, etc) or caught in a folding piece of equipment (stroller, folding chair, etc). Explosions and motor vehicle accidents seem to be the commonest causes for mutilating hand injuries in the older child. Explosions are unique in that they not only cause severe injuries, but also have components of both trauma and burns, thus rendering their care that much more challenging.

Nonaccidental injuries are uncommon but need to be kept in mind while evaluating any child with injuries. These types of injuries are more likely to be present on the cheeks, necks, genitals, and so on, and less likely to involve exposed areas such as the upper extremity.[6] In our experience, severe nonaccidental injuries of the upper extremity are more likely to be burns than any form of direct trauma. It is incumbent on the treating physician to be acutely aware of the possibility of these injuries and, if suspected, take appropriate measures to safeguard and protect the well-being of the child. This can involve immediate steps, such as separating the child from the offending adult, as well as long-term measures, such as notifying appropriate childhood protective and social service organizations.

Self-mutilating disorders are rare but can be devastating for the affected patient as well as parents. The best-known condition in this group is Lesch–Nyhan syndrome. This is inherited as an X-linked recessive condition and is caused by the deficiency of hypoxanthine guanine phosphoribosyl transferase. Features include mental retardation, hyperuricemia, and a tendency to self-mutilate. Patients are known to chew off various parts of their body, especially their digits (**Fig. 1**). Owing to the severity of mental retardation, continued tendency to self-mutilate as well as limited life expectancy, Lesch–Nyhan syndrome is one of the few mutilating conditions of the hand in a child where reconstructive procedures are contraindicated. Management is limited to controlling infection and revision amputation of affected digits.

Preservation, Care, and Transportation of Amputated Parts

It is imperative that amputated parts be preserved appropriately and transported rapidly to a center with microsurgical capability. Our center, which pioneered the repair of digital vessels under the late Harold Kleinert, has over the last 6 decades ensured that all emergency rooms within our catchment area are furnished with kits for this very purpose (**Fig. 2**). These comprehensive kits contain all material

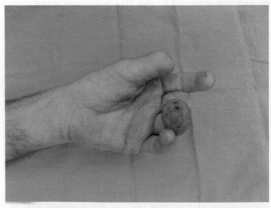

Fig. 1. A patient with Lesch-Nyan syndrome demonstrating multiple amputated digits owing to self-mutilation. The most recent injury is the infected long finger where recent bite marks are clearly visible over the tip. (*Courtesy of* KleinertKutz Hand Care Center, Louisville, KY; with permission.)

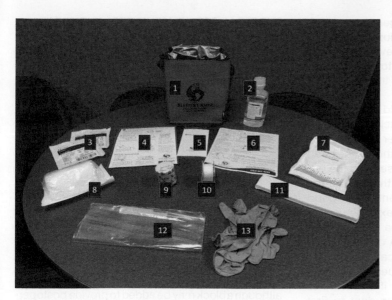

Fig. 2. Replantation kit with various items deemed necessary for correct preservation and transportation of an amputated part as well as injured limb. The various contents include (1) insulated kit, (2) sterile saline, (3) gauze pads, (4) instructions for correct packaging of an amputated part, (5) information brochure about replantation, (6) directions to our center, (7) cold pack (for placement on the injured limb; particularly useful to reduce warm ischemia as well as provide some pain relief, (8) gauze bandage roll, (9) elastic ace wrap, (10) adhesive tape, (11) Alumina-foam padded splint, (12) waterproof sealable plastic bags, and (13) gloves. (*Courtesy of* KleinertKutz Hand Care Center, Louisville, KY; with permission.)

required for proper preparation and packaging of an amputated part. They also have material that may be needed to dress and splint the injured limb. The kits also contain educational material about replantation, instructions about packaging the part, and directions to get to our center. In addition to emergency rooms, we have also provided these kits to the in-house medical facilities of large industries in the neighborhood. We have also ensured that all emergency room physicians and industrial medical staff are regularly educated and familiarized with procedures for recovery, preservation, and transportation of the amputated part as well as appropriate bandaging and dressing of the injured hand. A very important factor in this regard is to rely on compressive dressings and not tourniquets for control of bleeding. Although it is easy and hence tempting to apply a tourniquet, one cannot fail to remember that doing so creates an ischemic environment in the entire extremity, thus adversely affecting its survival and at the same time limiting the tourniquet time available for surgery. If a severely injured extremity is still attached to the body but devascularized, it cannot be preserved in ice. Consequently, it is now subject to warm ischemia, to which tissues are less tolerant. One way of mitigating this is to immobilize the extremity in a splint and then place a cold pack over it. Our replantation kit has provision for all of these eventualities.

The amputated part must first be wrapped in a moist dressing soaked in sterile saline or Ringer's lactate. This should then be placed in a waterproof plastic bag or container, which is then placed in a second larger bag or container that is filled with 3 parts ice and 1 part water. The whole package is then placed in an insulated bag for transportation.

It is important that the amputated part not be frozen. Water contracts till a temperature of 4°C is reached and then starts expanding; below this, a phenomenon known as anomalous expansion of water occurs. Consequently, if an amputated part were to be frozen, intracellular fluids could freeze and then expand, thus potentially rupturing cell membranes, leading to irreversible cell death. Alas, a solidly frozen part may not be suitable for replantation and unfortunately may have to be rejected.

INITIAL EVALUATION

Mutilating injuries by their very nature present unique challenges to the treating physician. The very cause of the injury is often a dramatic event that involves heavy machinery, automobiles, fire, or explosions. This provides an element of added psychological trauma to the injury that, because it affects the hand, is not just grotesque but very visibly so. Add into this mix the fact that such an injury involves a child, and we have a very serious social situation that the treating physician needs to confront even before getting down to the nitty gritty of managing the actual injury.

Anxious parents and a very scared and alarmed child are among the first things that one needs to be aware of when dealing with mutilating injuries in children. It is very important to quickly take command of the situation and to ensure that the parents are made to feel comfortable that their child is in good hands and will be taken care of. It is not uncommon for some parents to feel overprotective and hence seem overbearing to the hand surgeon. It takes tact and a calm but firm demeanor to handle such situations. We have found it useful if the parents are gently led away from the child during an examination to enable a tension-free environment. It may even be useful for another member of the team to sit with and talk to the parents while the main treating physician assesses the injury.

The initial assessment of a child with a mutilating injury must and should include a quick overall assessment to exclude other more serious life threatening injuries. Once this has been cleared, attention turns toward assessing the extremity. Experience has taught us that pain is the single most important impediment to a good physical examination. In this context, the usefulness of immediate local anesthesia for pain control cannot be overemphasized. A quick wrist or digital block can work wonders in calming the patient and thus make any subsequent evaluation that much more easier. However, if one were to use local anesthesia, it may be prudent to first assess for sensation in the digits. Static 2-point discrimination, assessed just distal to the distal interphalangeal crease, is the best way to document sensibility of a hand. Once this has been recorded, a local anesthetic block can be applied and further examination carried out under the umbrella of comfort that it provides the patient. The next system to be assessed is vascularity of the extremity. This dictates the urgency with which the patient needs to be moved into the operating room. Quite obviously, an avascular extremity, especially one in which the limb is still attached to the rest of the body and hence prone to warm ischemia, needs to be transported rapidly to the operating room. Once the nervous and vascular systems have been evaluated, radiographs can be obtained, ensuring at least 2 orthogonal views. Often pain precludes the ability to obtain true posteroanterior and lateral views and one may have to make do with oblique views. This apparent deficiency can be corrected subsequently in the operating room, where fluoroscopic evaluation can be carried out in greater detail under formal anesthesia.

Surgical consent obtained for a mutilating hand injury needs to be worded in general terms. It is best to avoid extremely specific terms, because it is not uncommon for initial assessments to be revised after evaluation in the operating room. It is also prudent to obtain consent for possible revision amputation of the affected digits or extremity as well as for possible vein, nerve, skin, and even bone grafts. An advantage in the case of a child is that the surgeon can subsequently obtain consent for additional procedures from parents, something that may not be so easy in an adult patient.

SURGICAL SEQUENCE IN REPLANTATION

Replantation can be defined as "a procedure in which everything a hand surgeon knows is done in 1 patient at the same time!"

The surgical sequence begins with preparation of the amputated part. The obvious advantage of doing so is that the team can begin working even before the patient is anesthetized or brought into the operating room. Sharp debridement is generally preferred and is carried out under loupe magnification or under the operating microscope. Arteries, nerves and veins are identified and tagged with 9-0 sutures. It is prudent to minimally dissect out these structures for tagging and not complete their final preparation, because that can be done later at the time of anastomosis. Sutures can be placed in tendons, as can K wires in the bone.

General anesthesia is preferred in children, although a block may be added to provide postoperative pain control. The bladder may be catheterized if it is felt that the procedure may take several hours. The amputation stump is prepared in a manner similar to the amputated part. Repair in finger replantation usually begins with bone fixation followed by repair of flexors, arteries, and nerves in that order. At this stage, the volar wound can be loosely closed and the hand turned around to proceed with repair of the extensor tendon and then veins.

Skeletal shortening can be performed to ensure better coaptation of bone as well as allow for tension-free repair of neurovascular structures and skin. K wires are our preferred method of fixation for digital replants; rigid methods of fixation such as plates and screws can be used for more proximal injuries. A special consideration in children is the presence of open physeal plates. Consequently, if at all possible, one needs to avoid crossing growth plates; if one must, smooth K wires are preferred to threaded devices to minimize injury and thus avoid future growth arrest. Notwithstanding all these precautions, it is still likely that the ischemic insult sustained at the time of injury may itself lead to premature physeal closure, a matter that is best explained to parents early on.

Flexor tendons are repaired immediately after skeletal fixation. Our preferred technique is to use a 6-strand core suture described from our center, followed by a running figure-of-8 epitendinous suture to ensure smooth gliding under the pulleys.[7,8] One may choose to repair just the flexor digitorum profundus alone to economize on time.

The next step involves repair of arteries. A question that one is often faced with involves selecting a suitable artery for repair. A study involving arterial injuries during World War II, reported loss of the hand in 1.6% of cases in whom the ulnar artery was ligated versus 5.1% loss of the extremity after ligating the radial artery.[9] A study conducted in our center specifically looked at which forearm artery contributed most blood flow to a specific digit using pulse volume plethysmography.[10] Of 1249 digits in 125 volunteers, only 5% were found to have ulnar artery dominance (ie, amplitude larger during radial artery compression) in all digits, and 28% were found to have complete radial artery dominance. Ulnar artery dominance in 3 or more digits was seen in 21.5% compared with 57% of radial artery dominance; 21.5% had equal dominance. Overall, 87% of thumbs, 70.5% of index, 60% of long, 52% of ring, and 52% of small fingers were found to be radial dominant (ie, the radial artery in the forearm—not the radial digital artery). Our experience over time has been that it is difficult to accurately predict dominance in any given situation. Hence, it is best to assess the status of vessels at the time of surgery and repair the best looking one. This is often the vessel that is least injured or the one with the greatest diameter. If possible and if time permits, it may be wise to repair both the ulnar and radial arteries.

An operating microscope or appropriate loupe magnification is necessary for repair of arteries to be carried out after proper preparation of vessel ends. The late Bob Acland, a pioneer in the field of microsurgery and founder of the Microsurgery Training Program in Louisville famously stated, "Preparation is the only shortcut you'll ever need to take" (R Acland, personal communication, 2003). He had these words literally carved in stone on a plaque that was prominently displayed in our microlaboratory to imprint its importance upon young trainees! Having suitably prepared the vessels, it is imperative that a tension-free repair be performed. The surgeon should readily opt for an interposition vein graft if the slightest doubt exists regarding tension at the repair site. Manipulating adjacent joints and placing them in extreme flexion to achieve primary end-to-end repairs is not done. A useful way to judge tension at the repair site is to place 1 or 2 coapting 9-0 sutures and then taking the finger through its full range of movement. Gapping of the anastomotic site is indicative of excessive tension and dictates need for interposition vein grafting.

On occasion, one may encounter a situation wherein the radial digital artery may be acceptable for anastomosis proximally and the ulnar digital artery suitable distally or vice versa. In such circumstances, a cross-anastomosis may have to be performed (**Fig. 3**). If ever the surgeon has to resort to such a technique, it is important to prominently record this in the operative notes for future reference. Often, these patients may need secondary surgical procedures such as tenolysis at a later date during

which the cross-anastomosed artery may be in danger of injury unless special care is taken.

Sometimes, the injury may have created a segmental defect in the vessels as well as covering soft tissues. In such cases, a flow through skin flap can be harvested along with an underlying subcutaneous vein and used to successfully bridge the defect in the vessel as well as the overlying skin (**Fig. 4**).

On rare occasions, especially those in which vein grafts may have to be used, one may encounter significant size discrepancies between vessels. Various methods have been described to overcome this. Small differences can be overcome using the halving technique, whereby 2 initial sutures are placed at 180° to each other and subsequent anastomosing sutures are placed at the midpoints between preceding sutures, thus equitably redistributing the size mismatch over the entire circumferences of the vessels. If the mismatch is greater, an oblique cut can be made in the smaller of the 2 vessels thus creating an opening that matches the size of the larger vessel, enabling anastomosis (**Fig. 5**). In contrast, the larger vessel can sometimes be trimmed and "funneled" down to reduce its end diameter thus enabling a direct end-to-end anastomosis (**Fig. 6**). In the rare circumstance when none of these are feasible, we have described a few other methods that may be used using vein grafts.[11]

Once the arteries and nerves are repaired, the volar wound can be closed loosely and the hand turned around for repair of the dorsal structures. The extensor tendons are first repaired, followed by veins. It is best to repair at least 2 veins for each artery that has been anastomosed. If adequate veins are not available, a vein graft may have to be used or, on occasion, a reversed cross-finger flap can be brought in from an adjacent digit to cover the deficit. In cases of replantations, it is our practice as a matter of routine to make a small fish-mouth incision at the tip of the finger at the time of surgery to decompress the digit and consequently reduce the load on repaired veins. This is kept open for 24 to 48 hours and allowed to bleed. Heparin-soaked pledgets are placed over the fingertip to prevent clotting of blood over the fish-mouth incision. We have used this method in the case of very distal replants where good veins are often unavailable for repair (**Fig. 7**). This step is not necessary in cases of revascularization where native veins are intact.

Tension-free closure of skin is the last and most important step. If necessary, relaxing z-plasties can be made to reduce a circumferential tightening around the extremity. In cases of macroreplants and revascularizations, proximal to the wrist, we routinely perform a prophylactic fasciotomy (**Fig. 8**).

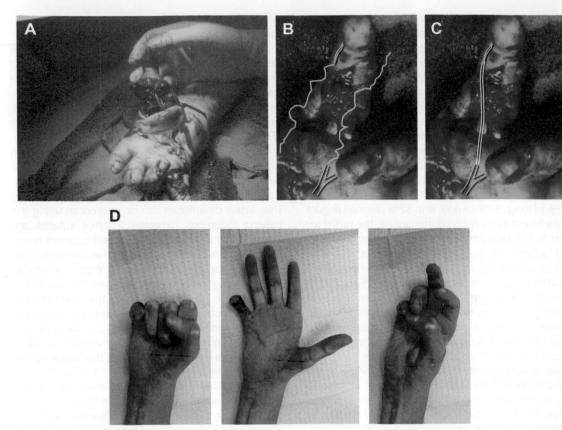

Fig. 3. A 12-year-old child sustained a firecracker explosion injury to his right hand. The thumb and small finger were devascularized and nearly amputated (*A*). It was possible to revascularize the thumb by direct anastomosis of the vessels. However, in the small finger, a small stump of the ulnar digital artery was available distally and a stump of the radial digital artery available proximally, with the rest of the vessels completely avulsed and damaged (*B*). A cross-anastomosis was performed using a vein graft (*C*). At final follow-up, the thumb survived completely and the small finger could be salvaged to a level just beyond the distal interphalangeal joint. The patient had a good range of movement and full return to function (*D*). (*Courtesy of* KleinertKutz Hand Care Center, Louisville, KY; with permission.)

POSTOPERATIVE CARE

Most hospitals do not have a dedicated hand floor available for children. This is the same in the case of our practice wherein we have a floor with trained nurses dedicated for the care of adult replants and revascularizations, but not one for children. Consequently, it may be necessary to admit the child to an intensive care unit (ICU) or an intermediate care unit rather than to a regular pediatric

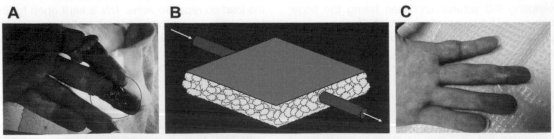

Fig. 4. A patient with a table saw injury was noted to have a devascularized digit with a segmental loss of the arteries along with a missing chunk of skin and subcutaneous tissue (*circle*) (*A*). A flow through flap was harvested along with a subcutaneous vein and surrounding fat (*B*, diagrammatic representation). This was then inset into the defect, successfully providing a bridge for the vascular and skin defect (*arrow*) (*C*). (*Courtesy of* Kleinert-Kutz Hand Care Center, Louisville, KY; with permission.)

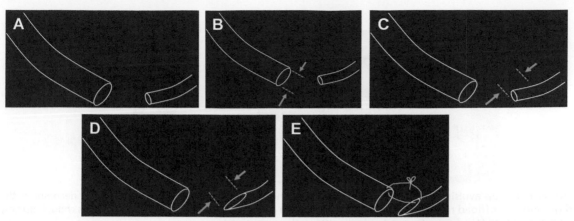

Fig. 5. Mismatched vessels with different diameters (*A*). Measure the diameter of the larger vessel (*B*) and then make an equivalent oblique cut in the smaller vessel (*C, D*). The 2 ends can then be approximated and anastomosed (*E*). (*Courtesy of* KleinertKutz Hand Care Center, Louisville, KY; with permission.)

surgical floor. This is necessitated by the fact that a replanted digit requires regular and around-the-clock monitoring. The surrounding temperature in the room needs to be kept warm (≥75°F).

We use thermocouple recordings to monitor the health of the digit. Temperatures are recorded at the exposed fingertip, every hour for the first 12 hours, and then spread out to every 4 hours provided the finger is doing well. A temperature decrease of greater than 3°C between an injured digit and an adjacent uninjured digit (or the opposite hand) is considered significant. Patients are routinely kept nil per os for the first 24 hours just in case they need to be brought back into the operating room for a reexploration. After that period, a regular diet is allowed except for

chocolates and caffeine. Smoking is strictly to be avoided and it behooves the surgeon to remember that this habit is not necessarily uncommon in children.

Here is a note of caution about care in an ICU setting that is unique to replants in children. It is very important for the ICU nursing staff to realize that the main component of postoperative care is "masterly inactivity" with the patient being disturbed as little as possible. The only regular activities necessary are thermocouple readings and changing of heparin pledgets. It is not necessary to monitor every single biological and biochemical parameter of this particular child, in contrast with the other sick and ill children who constitute the typical patients admitted to a pediatric ICU. This

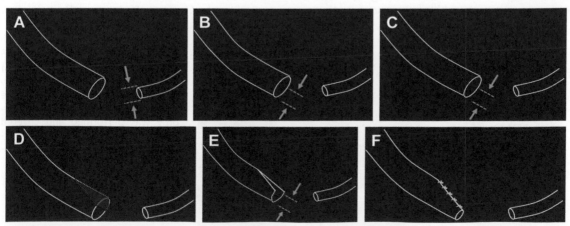

Fig. 6. Mismatched vessels can also be overcome by measuring the diameter of the smaller vessel (*A*), after which a corresponding size is marked out on the larger vessel (*B*). An oblique cut is then made in the larger vessel (*C*) after which the cut segment is excised (*D, E*). The obliquity is then sutured, thus funneling the larger vessel into a smaller diameter corresponding to the smaller vessel (*F*). (*Courtesy of* KleinertKutz Hand Care Center, Louisville, KY; with permission.)

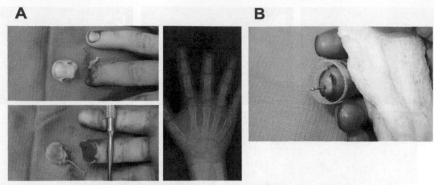

A   **B**

Fig. 7. Fingertip avulsion amputation in a child (*A*). Fish-mouth incision made over the pulp to decompress the digit and also offload repaired veins (*B*). Note also that a postoperative splint was not used in this child. (*Courtesy of* KleinertKutz Hand Care Center, Louisville, KY; with permission.)

has to be emphasized early on and the ICU team made aware of this fact. Another curious feature we have observed is the general level of interest that a replant arouses in an ICU. Because it is not very common to see children with replants, medical students, residents, and all staff members working in the ICU may be unduly curious and hence crowd around the child wanting to take a look. We have had to very firmly stop this practice of every person in the ICU "wanting to take a peek." Unnecessary handling of the replant can jeopardize its survival and this needs to be made clear early on.

Over the years we have found that postoperative splinting can be a problem in children, particularly very young ones. It used to be our practice in the past to routinely place replants in long arm casts. Care was taken to place such casts with the elbow flexed beyond 90° to reduce the chance of the child wriggling out of the cast (**Fig. 9**). Nonetheless, experience is a bitter pill, and over time we

have come to accept the fact there is probably no type of splint that a child will be unable to wriggle out of (**Fig. 10**)! This has led us to drastically reduce the amount of splinting not only after replants, but in young children in general. We prefer a well-padded dressing, with a simple dorsal block splint. In distal replants, we have abandoned the use of splints altogether in very young children without any adverse effects on outcomes (see **Fig. 7**).

Postoperatively, we routinely place a patient on antibiotics and appropriate analgesia. Anticoagulation is maintained by an intravenous infusion of heparin at a dose of 3 U/kg body weight per hour. This is maintained for the first 12 to 24 hours. If the replanted part is doing well, the dose is sequentially halved every 12 hours over the next 24 to 36 hours and then stopped altogether. The patient is then monitored for a further 12 to 24 hours and if the part remains viable, is considered fit for discharge. The use of

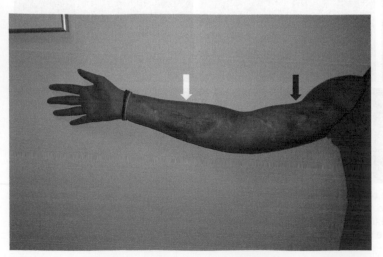

Fig. 8. Major limb revascularization in a 14-year-old child. The site of injury is marked with a black arrow and the white arrow points to the area where a prophylactic fasciotomy was performed and covered with a skin graft. (*Courtesy of* KleinertKutz Hand Care Center, Louisville, KY; with permission.)

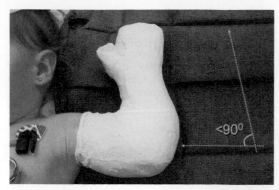

Fig. 9. Postoperative cast with the elbow flexed beyond 90° to reduce chances of the child wriggling out of the cast. (*Courtesy of* KleinertKutz Hand Care Center, Louisville, KY; with permission.)

low-molecular-weight dextran is to be avoided in children. Renal clearance may be inadequate, increasing the risk of renal failure as well as increasing the levels of fibrin degradation products in blood. By the same token, aspirin is to be avoided in young children to avoid the risk of Reye syndrome. If used in older children, oral aspirin is preferred to suppositories. A study revealed that the mean retention time for aspirin suppositories was about 4 hours and only about 60% of the drug was absorbed.[12]

CONTRAINDICATIONS TO REPLANTATION

One of the first contraindications to attempting replantation of an extremity is if there are other life-threatening injuries that obviously take precedence and hence preclude the extremity surgeons from operating on the child. Self-mutilating conditions such as Lesch–Nyhan syndrome are another

contraindication to any heroic reconstructive attempts (see **Fig. 1**).

Severe crushing and avulsion injuries may render tissues nonreconstructible. The presence of a "Chinese streak" on either side of a digit is a contraindication to attempting replantation. This sign suggests complete avulsion of all side branches from the digital arteries with subsequent leaking of blood from the avulsed vessel, forming a linear reddish-blue streak along the length of the digit (**Fig. 11**).

Prolonged ischemia is also a contraindication for replantation. This becomes particularly important in the case of larger replants. Another factor impacting survival is whether the ischemia was cold or warm. In general, digits can tolerate up to 4 hours of warm ischemia and up to 6 hours of cold ischemia. Larger parts, especially ones in which muscle tissue is present, can tolerate warm ischemia for about 2 to 3 hours and cold ischemia for about 4 hours. It is important to factor in surgical time as well into ones calculations, remembering that surgical time is essentially warm ischemia. Another useful test to determine feasibility of replantation in forearm or arm level amputations is the "thumb test." The surgeon attempts to passively move the thumb in the amputated part. If the thumb is found to be rigid and immobile, it suggests that rigor mortis has set in and the extremity is nonreplantable (Dr S Raja Sabapathy, personal communication, 2010).

ALTERNATIVES TO REPLANTATION

In situations where replantation is not possible, either owing to the presence of contraindications

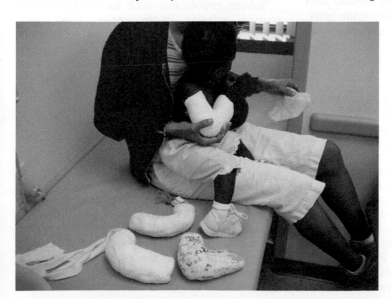

Fig. 10. Picture of a child in his fourth cast—the child managed to wriggle out of all the previous 3 casts, which the mother collected for posterity! (*Courtesy of* Kleinert-Kutz Hand Care Center, Louisville, KY; with permission.)

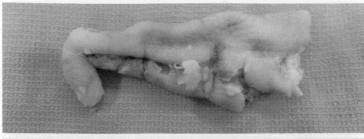
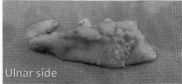
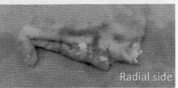

Ulnar side

Radial side

Fig. 11. Chinese streak sign seen on both the radial and ulnar sides of an avulsion amputation. The radial side has been magnified for clarity. (*Courtesy of* KleinertKutz Hand Care Center, Louisville, KY; with permission.)

or owing to the unavailability of adequate microsurgical expertise, alternative methods may have to be resorted to. The commonest method used is composite grafting. Reattaching the amputated part without microsurgical anastomosis of the vessels is a well-established practice, especially for tip amputations. The average survival of composite tissue grafts is about 24%. However, cooling the part for 72 hours has been known to improve survival rates to 91% and has been reported in fingertips as well as in the nose and ear.[13–15] The challenge in the hand is that placing the entire hand on a bag of ice can be very uncomfortable to adjacent uninjured digits and also cannot ensure that the operated digit stays in contact with the cooling surface. A method to overcome this hurdle using a syringe and surgical glove has been described.[16] Reducing its bulk while at the same time providing a better vascularized bed can also increase survival of the composite graft. Various techniques have been described to achieve this.[17–19]

PROGNOSIS

Overall, the survival of replantation in children is lesser than that in adults. There are 2 factors that principally contribute to this adverse outcome. The first factor is the extremely small caliber of vessels in children that, understandably, presents a significant surgical challenge. The second factor is the very nature of injury. It is more likely than not for a child to have sustained an amputation because of the finger getting caught in a window, door, or stroller. Consequently, the injury is most often a crush avulsion, which in turn adversely affects outcomes. A study done in our center revealed that survival of replants after clean guillotine amputations was around 94%. This

decreased to 80% in crush injuries and further decreased to 74% in avulsion amputations.[4]

SECONDARY PROCEDURES

Quite often, mutilating injuries in children may not be amenable to immediate complete repair. In addition, some injuries, although not resulting in amputation of an extremity, can leave the child with significant tissue deficits. Such injuries may require secondary reconstructive procedures with pedicled or free tissue transfer (**Fig. 12**). If the hand is very severely injured, the surgeon may be faced with the situation of being able to save only a few digits. In such cases, tissue can sometimes be harvested from the nonsalvageable digits and used for bone, skin, vessel, and nerve grafts (**Fig. 13**).

Salvage procedures such as toe transfers to replace missing digits have been well-documented in literature. After the world's first successful hand transplantation, which was done in our center in 1099, this procedure is also gaining widespread acceptance for reconstruction of amputated extremities. It, however, remains a procedure that is considered experimental and is hence confined to a few large centers around the world.

BURNS

Burns contribute to a significant number of mutilating injuries of the hand, especially in children. The commonest causes are scalds when the child accidentally dips his or her hand into a vessel containing a hot liquid. Another mechanism of injury in a child is accidentally placing the hands on a hot stovetop.

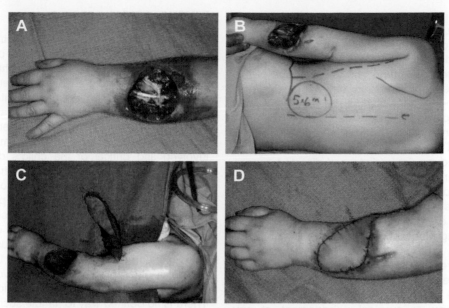

Fig. 12. A child presented with a significant soft tissue defect on the dorsum of the forearm (*A*). A paraspinal pedicled flap was designed to correspond to the size of the defect along with a proximal tail (*B*). This was then elevated on its pedicle and tunneled into the forearm (*C*) and was successfully used to cover the defect (*D*). (*Courtesy of* Kleinert-Kutz Hand Care Center, Louisville, KY; with permission.)

One needs to be acutely aware of the possibility of abuse and nonaccidental trauma when dealing with burns in children. The slightest doubt in this regard needs to be taken seriously and is probably best dealt with by notifying appropriate child protective services.

Classical teaching recommends aggressive debridement of burns with removal of blisters

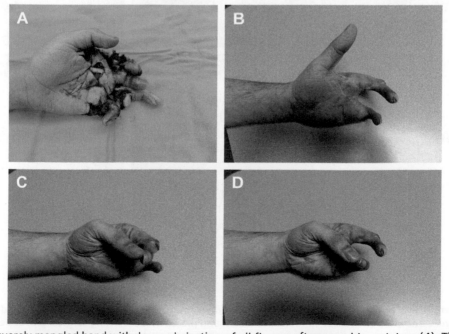

Fig. 13. A severely mangled hand with devascularization of all fingers after a machinery injury (*A*). The long and ring fingers were deemed unsalvageable but were used to obtain arterial grafts and skin grafts to reconstruct the index and small fingers (*B*). At final follow-up, the patient demonstrated good pulp-to-pulp opposition in both the reconstructed digits (*C, D*). (*Courtesy of* KleinertKutz Hand Care Center, Louisville, KY; with permission.)

and potential eschars followed by the application of silver sulfadiazine cream and an occlusive dressing. Compression garments have also been recommended. Our approach to burns has drastically changed over time and involves use of the glove–gauze regimen.[20] In this technique, the burned hand is anointed with silver sulfadiazine cream and placed in an oversized glove. No surgical debridement is carried out and all blisters are left intact. The mother or the child (if old enough) is instructed on immediate self-directed range-of-movement and stretching exercises. The gloves are changed twice daily. At each glove change, the hand is washed gently with an antibacterial soap, allowed to dry, and then reanointed with cream before being placed back in a glove. If significant maceration is noted, the hand may be wrapped in gauze dressing for the night. It is surprising to note how easily a child adapts to this method and to date not a single child has required formal physiotherapy or surgical debridement of any sort. Full range of movement with no scar contractures has been seen in all children treated by this method so far (**Fig. 14**).

PSYCHOLOGICAL ASPECTS

As alluded to earlier in this paper, a mutilating hand injury in a child can a have significant psychological impact. This not only affects the child, but can also have devastating effects on parents, guardians, and the family as a whole. Parental guilt can have unintended consequences. It has been reported that parents can often transfer their guilt to health care workers by becoming overly involved and critical of the child's care.[21] Our experience has further taught us that often 1 parent may have been involved in some way in the injury, as can happen if a child is playing with fireworks or operating a piece of machinery with 1 parent. In such situations, it is not uncommon for parents to vent their anger and frustration toward one another in the presence of the treating physician. Such problems can only worsen if the child happens to come from a divided family. There is no defined way to handle such situations and can hence place significant strain on medical personnel. One may have to adopt a kind but firm demeanor in these circumstances.

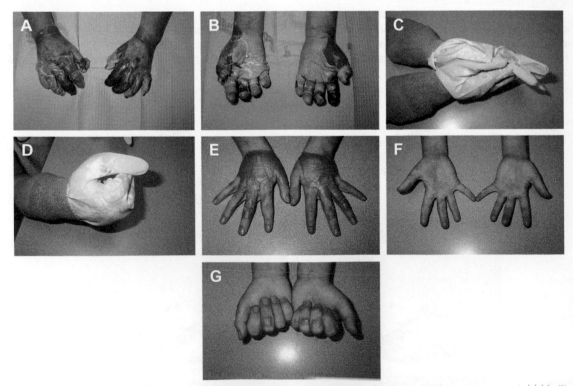

Fig. 14. Severe scalds can be seen on both the dorsal and volar aspects of both hands in a 5-year-old child (*A, B*). The hands were anointed with silver sulfadiazine cream and placed in loose fitting surgical gloves per the glove–gauze regimen. Immediate self-directed range-of-movement and stretching exercises were commenced; the child can be seen doing his own exercises (*C, D*). No surgical procedures of any kind were performed at any stage. At final follow-up, both hands had completely healed with no scar contractures and full range-of-movement was obtained in all fingers (*E–G*). (*Courtesy of* KleinertKutz Hand Care Center, Louisville, KY; with permission.)

Counseling can be of great benefit, but it is not an easy task to convince parents or guardians of the need to actually seek it. Our success in obtaining psychological intervention has been mixed at best.

SUMMARY

Mutilating injuries pose a challenge to any treating physician. Of all bodily injuries, hand injuries are extremely visible and particularly if occurring in a child bring with them added challenges of alarm, fear, guilt and other psychosocial factors that are beyond the control of a hand surgeon.

Care of the injured hand begins with education of emergency room personnel to ensure proper preservation and dispatch of amputated parts. Once received at the treating facility, a systematic planned approach, enforced by an experienced team can add significantly to bettering outcomes. A good physical therapy unit, trained in the care complex hand problems is absolutely essential and its contribution to results is to say the least, invaluable. The chances of satisfactory outcome are further enhanced by an early and thorough discussion with parents regarding expected outcomes and expected future reconstructive procedures.

Treating a child with a mutilating hand injury can, at the time, be an emotionally draining experience. But in the end, nothing can be more rewarding that the sight of a big smile on the face of a young boy who returns to your clinic to let you know that he has now returned to playing sports or a young lady who comes in to proudly display her first driver's license!

REFERENCES

1. Thirkannad S. Pediatric hand injuries. Chapter 15. In: Fallat ME, Roution GW, editors. Pediatric trauma manual. Kosair Childrens Hospital; 2013. p. 313-29.
2. Borse NN, Gilchrist J, Dellinger AM, et al. CDC Childhood Injury Report: Patterns of Unintentional Injuries among 0 -19 Year Olds in the United States, 2000-2006. Atlanta (GA): Centers for Disease Control and Prevention, National Center for Injury Prevention and Control; 2008.
3. National Center for Injury Protection and Control. WISQARS online nonfatal injury reports. Atlanta (GA): Centers for Disease Control and Prevention, National Center for Injury Prevention and Control; 2014.
4. Jaeger SH, Tsai TM, Kleinert HE. Upper extremity replantation in children. Orthop Clin North Am 1981;12(4):897-907.
5. Baker GL, Kleinert JM. Digit replantation in infants and young children: determinants of survival. Plast Reconstr Surg 1994;94(1):139-45.
6. Paul AR, Adamo MA. Non-accidental trauma in pediatric patients: a review of epidemiology, pathophysiology, diagnosis and treatment. Transl Pediatr 2014;3(3):195-207.
7. Gill RS, Lim BH, Shatford RA, et al. A comparative analysis of the six-strand double-loop flexor tendon repair and three other techniques: a human cadaveric study. J Hand Surg Am 1999;24(6): 1315-22 [Erratum appears in J Hand Surg Am 2000;25(3):590].
8. Silfverskiöld KL, Andersson CH. Two new methods of tendon repair: an in vitro evaluation of tensile strength and gap formation. J Hand Surg Am 1993;18(1):58-65.
9. Debakey ME, Simeone FA. Battle injuries of the arteries in world war II: an analysis of 2471 cases. Ann Surg 1946;123(4):534-79.
10. Kleinert JM, Fleming SG, Abel CS, et al. Radial and ulnar artery dominance in normal digits. J Hand Surg Am 1989;14(3):504-8.
11. Turker T, Tsai TM, Thirkannad S. Size discrepancy in vessels during microvascular anastomosis: two techniques to overcome this problem. Hand Surg 2012;17(3):413-7.
12. Nowak MM, Brundhofer B, Gibaldi M. Rectal absorption from aspirin suppositories in children and adults. Pediatrics 1974;54(1):23-6.
13. Heistein JB, Cook PA. Factors affecting composite graft survival in digital tip amputations. Ann Plast Surg 2003;50(3):299-303.
14. Hirasé Y. Postoperative cooling enhances composite graft survival in nasal-alar and fingertip reconstruction. Br J Plast Surg 1993; 46(8):707-11.
15. Chandawarkar RY, Cervino AL, Wells MD. Reconstruction of nasal defects using modified composite grafts. Br J Plast Surg 2003;56(1): 26-32.
16. Sunil TM. A technique for postoperative cooling after composite grafting of the fingertip. Tech Hand Up Extrem Surg 2006;10(2):118-9.
17. Dubert T, Houimli S, Valenti P, et al. Very distal finger amputations: replantation or "reposition-flap" repair? J Hand Surg Br 1997;22(3): 353-8.
18. Netscher DT, Meade RA. Reconstruction of fingertip amputations with full-thickness perionychial grafts from the retained part and local flaps. Plast Reconstr Surg 1999;104(6):1705-12.
19. Lee SM, Rahman MF, Thirkannad S. Combination V-Y advancement flap and composite graft for reconstruction of an amputated fingertip. Hand Surg 2012;17(1):145-9.
20. Coffey MJ, Thirkannad SM. Glove-gauze regimen for the management of hand burns. Tech Hand Up Extrem Surg 2009;13(1):4-6.
21. Buncke GM, Buntic RF, Romeo O. Pediatric mutilating hand injuries [review]. Hand Clin 2003;19(1): 121-31.

Skin Coverage Considerations in a Mutilating Hand Injury

Kyungjin Lee, MD, Siyoung Roh, MD, Dongchul Lee, MD, Jinsoo Kim, MD*

KEYWORDS

- Hand • Microsurgery • Free flap • Reconstruction

KEY POINTS

- Investigators believe that free tissue transfer is the most suitable way of providing a soft tissue cover in a mutilated hand.
- When free flap transfer is not technically possible or where microsurgery facility is not available, carefully planned regional or pedicled flaps work well.
- Hand surgeons must approach mutilating hand injuries with the recognition that no 2 injuries are ever the same.
- Should try to replace like with like tissue.
- Both function and aesthetics should be given consideration.

INTRODUCTION

The hand is a highly specialized organ with a complex mechanical structure. Because of the role that hand plays in manipulating objects, it is the most frequent site of trauma in the body and is subject to mutilation through various injury mechanisms. Such mutilating injuries never occur the same way, and each injury requires meticulous evaluation. Once all deficiencies in tissue are identified, the decision must be made as to which portions must be sacrificed or preserved to maximize functional recovery.[1]

When reconstructing a mutilated hand, the primary goal is to provide stable skin and soft tissue coverage. The secondary goals are to restore motor function, shape, and sensation to the hand. Del Piñal recommended the following criteria in defining the acceptable hand concept: a hand with 3 fingers of near normal length, near-normal PIP joint motion, good sensibility, and a functioning thumb.[2] Such guidelines are helpful in organizing a reconstructive plan. What constitutes a set of components for a functional hand can vary, however, according to race, gender, age, occupation, inclination, lifestyle, and hand dominance. In addition, it is difficult for a surgeon to consider all of the ramifications these variations hold for reconstructive priority. Because of this, the authors tend to fall back to the classic principle of restoring as much of natural function as possible.

To maximize the restoration of functions, the initial aim should be to preserve as much of the vital structures as possible, such as neurovascular structures, bone and joint, tendon, and intrinsic musculature. Early skin coverage is the best method of preserving these tissues and, therefore, should be in the foremost consideration during the initial encounter and primary intervention in the management of a mutilated hand.

Skin coverage can largely be divided between nonmicrosurgical and microsurgical options.[3]

Department of Plastic and Reconstructive Surgery, Gwang-Myeong Sung-Ae General Hospital, 36 Digital-ro, Gwangmyeong, Gyungki-do 423711, Korea
* Corresponding author.
E-mail address: drkim@korea.com

Hand Clin 32 (2016) 491–503
http://dx.doi.org/10.1016/j.hcl.2016.07.002
0749-0712/16/© 2016 Elsevier Inc. All rights reserved.

Nonmicrosurgical options include skin graft and various local flaps but find limited use in providing adequate coverage. Skin grafts cannot be used over exposed vital structures and can result in severe contracture. Local flaps or pedicled flaps allow coverage with composite tissue but are limited to specific skin territories. Most such local flaps were developed for specific tissue defects of predetermined size and location and are inappropriate for use in mutilated hands, in which further sacrifice of soft tissue only adds to the devastation of tissues. Although delayed reconstruction is well tolerated in the lower extremity, this is not the same for the hand.[4] Increasing the duration of immobilization can cause joint stiffness and tendon adhesion and makes an adverse effect for secondary procedure. Thus, the authors believe that early coverage using microsurgical free tissue transfer represents the best initial management of the mutilated hand. This article discusses options for free skin flap coverage of the mutilating hand.

FLAP SELECTION FOR HAND RESURFACING

Although advancement in microsurgical techniques have allowed a wide variety in free flap options, most instances of flap selection continue to be influenced by surgeon preference. Generally, the selection of a specific flap should reflect the following considerations: the size and depth of the tissue defect; injury mechanism; underlying structures, either exposed or requiring reconstruction; sensation; skin characteristics; donor-site morbidity; and the need for secondary procedure. Among these, the following specific issues must be addressed for a functional hand resurfacing:

1. Tissue thickness: the flap usually needs to be thin to allow for acceptable contour.
2. Sensation recovery: innervated flaps provide better outcomes.
3. Pliability: the flap needs to be pliable for 3-D resurfacing without impairment in motion.

4. Gliding capacity: the inner surface of the flap must be smooth to allow for tendon excursion.[5]

It is extremely difficult to identify a flap that satisfies all these requirements and each flap should be considered based on the characteristics of the skin according to the location of surface defect. Specialized surfaces are ideally replaced like with like tissue.

Skin characteristics differ significantly between dorsal and volar surfaces with inherent differences in physiologic role. The volar skin is composed of a thick layer of heavily cornified epithelial surface. The dermis is firmly attached to the underlying fibrous fascia and exhibits significant resistance to shearing force. The glabrous surface, although tough, provides tactile sensation. In contrast, the dorsal skin is thin and pliable, which allows for joint movement.[6,7] Superior restoration of function is accorded to reconstructions using flaps that most closely match the tissue being replaced. Because of this, the decision-making process should compare the pros and cons of each flap under consideration. At the authors' institution, the algorithm for mutilated hand management considers skin resurfacing options based on location-specific characteristics (**Fig. 1**).

DORSAL SKIN COVERAGE

The most significant characteristic of the dorsal skin is that it is thin and allows for significant stretching. From the reconstructive perspective, this property necessitates that dorsal surface defects must not be resurfaced with bulky, nonpliable tissue, where such flaps result in poor range of motion and aesthetic outcome. Most of the widely used fasciocutaneous free flaps do not satisfy this requirement and are only appropriate for use where a bulky flap is used to fill dead space and where it would not interfere with joint motion (**Fig. 2**).

Several options are available for thin-skin resurfacing. The free forearm yields a thin cutaneous flap, using either the radial or the ulnar artery as

Location / Size	Volar side	Dorsal side	Pulp
Small	Venous free flap ?	Facial flap with skin graft	Hypothenar flap
	Toe plantar flap		
			Second toe pulp flap
	Thenar (iRASP) flap	Various cutaneous flap with debulking	
Large	Medial plantar flap		Great toe pulp flap

Fig. 1. Algorithm of selecting the flap based on location of the defect. iRASP, innervated radial artery superficial palmar branch flap.

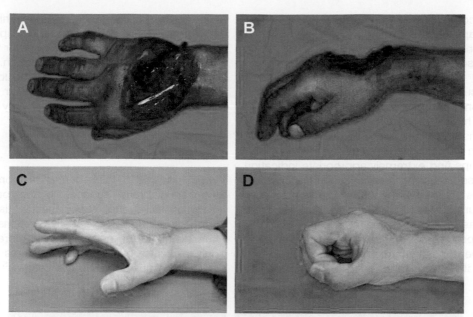

Fig. 2. Lateral arm free flap for a significant composite soft-tissue defect (*A, B*) in a 42-year-old patient who was injured by a hydraulic linkage. This defect was resurfaced using sensate lateral arm free flap. (*C, D*) At 5-year follow-up visit, the reconstructed hand maintains acceptable hand contour and sufficient range of motion.

pedicles. Unfortunately, these forearm flaps are still not as thin as the dorsal skin of the hand, and flap margin contracture can result in increasing bulkiness in the postoperative period. The hair growth, poor take of skin graft, and esthetic and functional donor-site morbidities are major disadvantages.[8,9]

Another option is to cover the dorsal defect with a cutaneous flap and defat or debulk the tissue in a secondary procedure. Even the thinnest of fasciocutaneous flaps contains a layer of subcutaneous fat and requires a secondary procedure to reduce the thickness of the fat layer or revise the contour of flap margins. The downside to this approach is the long delay between the primary and secondary operations, and aggressive defatting can adversely affect flap circulation and lead to skin necrosis. No matter how much fat is removed, such flaps can never be as thin as the original dorsal skin.

As much as early postoperative exercise is important to functional recovery, dorsal defects should be recovered using as thin a skin flap as possible at the time of the primary operation.[10,11] Cutaneous flaps can be immediately defatted during the flap-insetting stage of the initial operation. Dissection around the pedicle is difficult, however, and this makes for an irregular contour. Aggressive dissection is to be avoided around the pedicle. Flaps can be elevated along the superficial fascia plane to avoid the need for secondary debulking procedure altogether.[12] Despite various methods for reducing flap thickness, the authors are of the opinion that, fundamentally, cutaneous free flaps cannot provide satisfactory hand contour.

At the authors' institution, most dorsal surface defects are covered with free fascial flaps with secondary split-thickness skin graft, which represents the thinnest resurfacing option. The first report on the use of a free fascial flap was made in 1990 by Smith. A subsequent report by Yousif and colleagues[13] popularized the use of lateral arm fascial free flap. Fascial flaps can be raised from many locations (radial forearm, temporoparietal, serratus anterior, lateral arm, dorsal ulnar forearm, and anterolateral thigh).[14-20] Among these, the authors' most frequently used free fascia flaps are lateral arm and anterolateral thigh fascial flaps.

The lateral arm fascia flap shares many of the advantages of the lateral arm cutaneous flap, including the ability to cover wide defects. The flap demonstrates robust axial perfusion through the suprafascial vascular network. The flap is raised with the posterior radial collateral artery as the center pedicle and can combine anterior skin (over biceps, brachialis, and brachioradialis) and posterior skin (over triceps) for flap dimensions up to 9 cm × 12 cm.[21,22] The anterolateral thigh can yield even larger fascia envelope with longer vascular pedicle.

Most common arguments against the use of fascial flaps revolve around limited flap size, the risk of tendon adhesion, or contracture from skin graft. Fascial flap is extremely pliable, however, and can cover complex surface defects. The smooth surface of fascia facilitates smooth gliding of tendon and minimizes the risk of adhesion (**Fig. 3**). This is an advantage unique to fascial flaps for reconstruction of the dorsum where tendon excursion is extremely relevant. Because of this, fascial flaps find extremely appropriate indication for exposed tendons and for situations in which transfer is planned in the future. Problematic scar contracture has yet to be reported for skin graft, which was placed over free fascial flap.[23]

It is important to minimize morbidity at the donor site. Patient dissatisfaction can be compounded by operative scar and become hypertrophied over conspicuous areas of the body. This is relevant at the donor site of cutaneous flaps, where primary closure inevitably results in scar widening and hypertrophy from increased tension. The use of skin graft leaves a highly conspicuous scar. Aesthetically, fascial flaps are superior because they do not leave hypertrophied or overly conspicuous scars (**Fig. 4**).

VOLAR SKIN COVERAGE

Volar skin has a thick dermis that provides a tougher glabrous surface. In the palm, the glabrous skin and subcutaneous tissue are perfectly adapted to serve the prehensile function.[24] Defects of the palmar skin represent not only exposure of functional structures but also loss of the unique tissue architecture.[5] Maximal

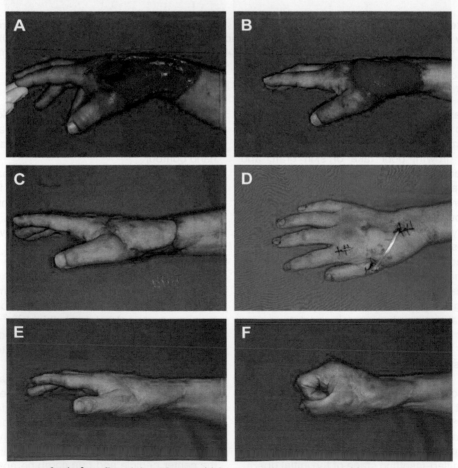

Fig. 3. Lateral arm fascia free flap. (*A*) A 58-year-old female patient was injured by a condenser motor with resulting tissue defect in the dorsal skin and extensor tendons. (*B*) The defect was covered with lateral arm fascia free flap. Split-thickness skin graft was applied at 2 weeks later. (*C*) At 5 months after the initial operation, the dorsal surface has an acceptable contour. (*D*) Extensor indicis proprius was transferred for extensor pollicis longus reconstruction in the layer below the fascial surface of the flap. (*E, F*) At 6-month follow-up from tendon transfer operation, the thumb can move through the full range of motion.

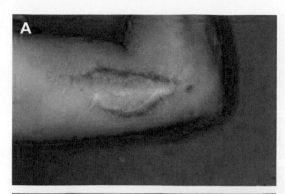

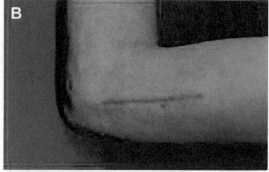

Fig. 4. A comparison of donor-site scar. (A) This cutaneous flap donor site could not be closed primarily. Despite the use of skin graft, the scar is wide and hypertrophic change. (B) In contrast, the donor-site scar is relatively inconspicuous where only the fascia was harvested.

functional recovery is possible only by replacing the lost tissue with glabrous skin. No donor source exists, however, for large defects of glabrous skin, and, in such cases, the reconstruction must resort to nonglabrous cutaneous flaps. If the defect is not in the web space, the flap does not require extensive thinning. In certain contexts (ie, significant dead space or need for grasp function), tissue volume is even desirable. In obese patients, abundance of subcutaneous fat can be a problem, and fascial free flap with skin graft represents a

good alternative. Compared with the dorsum, however, fascial flap with skin graft represents significant risk of contracture and color mismatch (**Fig. 5**). Wherever possible, the authors recommend neurosensate fasciocutaneous flap for volar surface coverage because of surface durability, soft tissue padding, and sensation.

Since the first report by Yoshimura and colleagues[25] in 1987, many surgeons have used venous free flap to cover small defects of the hand. Venous flap is a flow-through free flap and can be classified into 3 anastomotic types: artery to artery, artery to vein, and vein to vein. The flap incorporates afferent and efferent veins and can be used to reconstruct missing portions of artery or vein in the defect. In defects with missing vessel segments, venous flaps can provide both the coverage of soft tissue as well as revascularization of the distal tissue.[26] The flap is superficial and thin. It can be harvested quickly and does not require sacrifice of an arterial pedicle at the donor site.[27] Venous flaps lack a fascial layer, however, and are thus mechanically unrobust. Volume atrophy is difficult to estimate, and sensory recovery is poor. More importantly, venous congestion and edema in the early postoperative period can develop into flap necrosis, and this unpredictable nature of venous flap is what offsets many of its advantages.

The best alternative tissue for the volar skin of the hand is skin from other portions of the volar surface and from the plantar surface. Various flaps have incorporated glabrous tissues and can be classified according to recipient footprint. This discussion focuses on resurfacing of volar defects other than fingertips; the latter is discussed separately in a later section.

For small volar defects, the recommended option is toe plantar flap (**Fig. 6**).[28] It is a neurosensate flap and commonly used to cover small defects of the proximal surface of digits. The flap pedicle can be used as interposition graft for

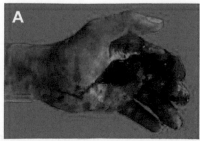

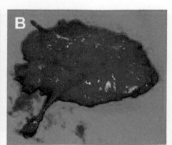

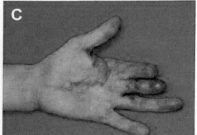

Fig. 5. Coverage of volar surface defect. (A) This left hand has significant loss of volar soft tissue. (B) This lateral arm fascia free flap was insetted into the defect. A split-thickness skin graft was applied at a secondary operation. (C) The palm skin is showed thin. Contracture and skin discoloration, however, is obvious.

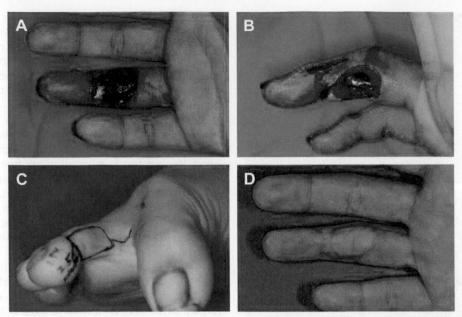

Fig. 6. Toe plantar free flap. (*A, B*) This patient had volar surface of the right ring finger caught in a chain with resultant soft tissue defect and loss of neurovascular continuity on the radial side. (*C*) The plantar flap was taken from the second right toe. The flap was harvested as a flow-through flap and was used for neurovascular interposition. (*D*) At 1-year follow-up visit, the flap matches the surrounding volar tissue in color with continuity of crease.

neurovascular bundle injury. The second toe is most commonly used to decrease donor-site morbidity, and the harvested flap can be designed to incorporate the volar crease over the interphalangeal joint. Often, the donor site cannot be closed primarily and may require skin graft.[29]

Moderately sized volar defect can be resurfaced using the free thenar flap (**Fig. 7**). This flap was first reported by Kamei and colleagues[30] in 1993. Subsequent to this, the study by Omokawa and colleagues[31] provided an improved understanding into the anatomy of thenar structure and popularized the thenar free flap as a good option for volar skin coverage. The indication for this flap was limited to digital soft tissue defect, and some investigators consider local or island homodigital or heterodigital flap just as good a solution without the trouble of microanastomosis.[32] The authors believe, however, that thenar flaps are options superior to local flaps for volar defects at the distal level. The thenar area has an abundance of sensory receptors, and multiple cutaneous nerve branches can be incorporated at the time of harvest. As such, sensory recovery of this flap appears above par for glabrous tissue free flaps. An average dimension of 2.4 cm × 7.8 cm has been reported in the past, with primary closure of donor site possible in most cases.[33] An additional advantage is that the flap can be harvested within the same operative field.

For large volar surface defects, the plantar surface represents the only viable option for

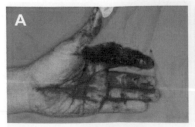
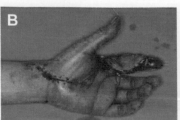
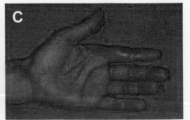

Fig. 7. Free thenar flap. (*A*) A 54-year-old male patient was injured by a saw-toothed wheel. The left index finger shows signs of severe crushing injury with soft tissue defect. (*B*) An emergency operation was performed to cover the defect using innervated radial artery superficial branch perforator flap (free thenar flap). (*C*) At 8-month follow-up visit, the index finger maintains a thin and durable volar surface.

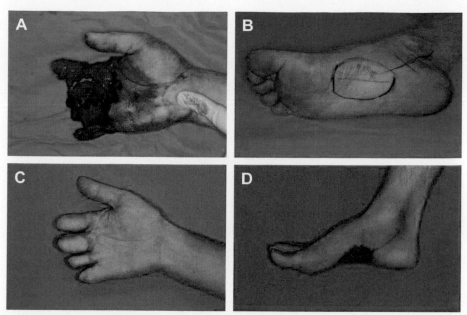

Fig. 8. Medial plantar free flap. (*A*) This 47-year-old man was injured by a rolling mill with resultant mutilation of the hand down to the metacarpal level. (*B*) A medial plantar free flap was elevated for damage-control coverage of the exposed surface. (*C*) At 2-year follow-up, the volar surface demonstrates acceptable skin color and texture. (*D*) The donor site was managed with split-thickness skin graft.

resurfacing with glabrous skin. Plantar skin has the tissue characteristics extremely close to palmar skin and matches the physical function. Plantar skin flap was first described by Shanahan and Gingrass[34] and was used to cover soft tissue defects of the heel. The largest skin tissue can be harvest in the non–weight-bearing, medial plantar surface, and, because of this, the flap is referred to as medial plantar free flap or instep free flap[35] (**Fig. 8**). The flap pedicle is a perforator of the medial plantar artery and venae comitantes. Because the flap sacrifices only the superficial portion of the plantar vascular arcade, the vascular supply to the plantar muscle is preserved. It can be harvested as a sensate flap by incorporating medial plantar nerve. Up to 9 cm ×10 cm of flap

dimensions are possible, which is large enough to resurface nearly all of the palmar skin.

Harvesting a large area of plantar skin necessitates skin graft at the donor site. Donor-site morbidities include pain, gait changes, discomfort, and difficulty wearing normal footwear. A portion of these morbidities can be mitigated by using full-thickness skin graft instead of split-thickness skin graft.[36]

PULP COVERAGE

In the management of volar surface defect, fingertip (pulp) defects requires special consideration. The soft tissue used to reconstruct fingertip must have thick glabrous skin with adequate padding. Above all, the protective sensation

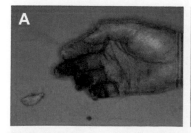
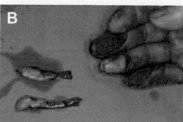
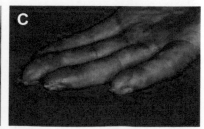

Fig. 9. Multiple toe pulp free flap. (*A*) A 47-year-old male patient was injured by a rolling mill with resultant fingertip defect in third, fourth, and fifth digits of the right hand. The amputated soft tissue had been recovered only for the ring finger. (*B*) The ring fingertip was replanted. Second toe pulp flaps were harvested from second toes bilaterally. (*C*) At 8-month follow-up visit, the second toe pulp fingertip has contour similar to that of the uninjured index finger and that also of the replanted ring fingertip.

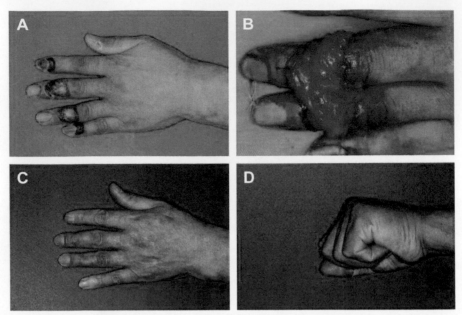

Fig. 10. Anterolateral thigh fascia free flap for finger dorsum. (*A*) A 56-year-old male patient was injured by a heated press with thermal-crush injury to the dorsum of multiple digits and resultant exposure of extensor tendons. (*B*) The defects over the third and fourth digits were covered by a single anterolateral thigh fascia free flap. The bridge flap was subsequently divided and covered with skin grafts. (*C*, *D*) At 8-year follow-up visit, appearance and function remain satisfactory for resurfaced digits.

must be restored. The magnitude of the problem represented by fingertip defect is demonstrated by the wide spectrum of solution offered in the literature. Reconstructive options that allow for satisfactory recovery of sensation include V-Y advancement flap,[37,38] neurovascular pedicled flap,[39] and sensate free tissue transfer. Among these, the reconstructive option with the least

amount of donor-site morbidity and the highest degree of tissue matching is free tissue transfer of toe pulp.[40] Toe pulp flaps are taken from either the big toe or the second toe. A portion of the pulp tissues is taken as to allow for primary closure of donor site. The constant anatomy of neurovascular bundle and subcutaneous vein allow for trouble-free harvest.

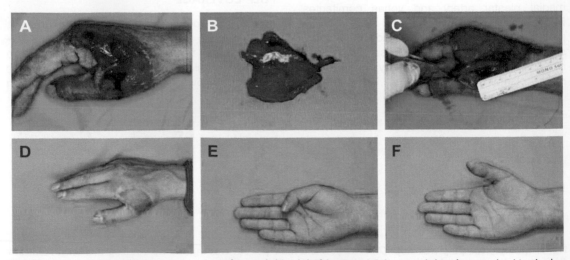

Fig. 11. Simultaneous reconstruction of tendon and skin. (*A*) This tangential-vector injury has resulted in the loss of soft tissue and tendon of right thumb extensor mechanism. (*B*) This tendofascial flap was harvested from the right lateral arm. (*C*) The vascularized tendon was placed as an interposition graft. (*D–F*) At 7-month follow-up, the right thumb demonstrates good range of motion with satisfactory contour.

The medial plantar skin can be used as a donor site, but the process of flap harvest is laborious. The flap does not easily conform to the convex contour of the fingertip. Patient satisfaction is sometimes low because of painful scar.[41,42] The skin from hypothenar eminence also has texture similar to fingertip skin and offers the advantage of single operative field.[43,44] It is difficult, however, to obtain a neurosensate flap, and donor-site scar can cause discomfort when using writing instruments or computer mouse.

Multiple pulp defects can be covered with a single large flap in a bridge pattern, but such an approach requires secondary division. The temporary syndactyly interferes with early rehabilitation. In such situations, multiple toe pulp flaps can be taken from big toes and second toes (**Fig. 9**). In the authors' review of second toe pulp flap donor-site morbidity, long-term follow-up has revealed that most patients did not experience any painful scars that limited daily activity.[45]

DIGITAL SKIN COVERAGE

Coverage of digital surface often requires wrap-around technique.[4] Reconstructive planning of digital skin coverage should reflect whether more of the dorsal or volar tissue is missing. Because digital skin does not require much laxity, the main strategy for resurfacing the finger should revolve around the provision of thin skin layer to minimize the risk of contracture or stiffness.[46] In the absence of tendon or bone exposure, either split-thickness or full-thickness skin graft can provide adequate coverage. Mutilating injury rarely spares the soft tissue, however, to the extent that the underlying skeletal system is not exposed. As such, skin grafts find little indication in mutilating injury, and vascularized tissue is used to cover most cases of mutilated digits.

Flap coverage for dorsal surface of digits do not differ significantly from flaps used for hand dorsum. The main difference is that even though the dorsal surface of digits does not have as much tendon excursion, the wider contact surface makes tendon adhesion more likely occurrence over the finger extensor surface. Even the slightest of bulkiness results in an unacceptable appearance and can inhibit full range of motion. Coverage with thin skin at primary operation is important in decreasing the immobilization period and, consequently, joint stiffness. When all these factors are considered, the dorsal surface of digits is most appropriately reconstructed using fascia free flap with skin graft. This solution is all the more applicable in the case of severe crushing injury, where

dorsal surfaces must be resurfaced over multiple digits (**Fig. 10**).

ASSOCIATED INJURY

Soft tissue defects are often accompanied by loss of deeper underlying tissue in mutilating injuries. Skin coverage is the foremost goal, but defects other than skin should also be reconstructed if possible at the time of damage control operation. Tendon injury is a common finding during the evaluation of a mutilated hand. Flexor tendons are

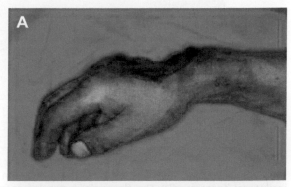

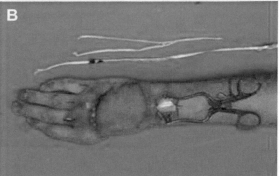

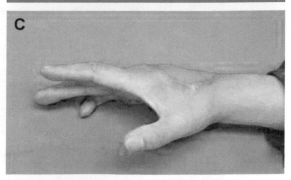

Fig. 12. Delayed reconstruction of multiple tendon injuries. (*A*) Preoperative photograph of a dorsal soft tissue injury with multiple extensor tendon involvement. The soft tissue defect was covered with a fasciocutaneous free flap. (*B*) Intraoperative photograph at the time of delayed tendon reconstruction using plantaris tendon. (*C*) Postoperative functional evaluation demonstrates satisfactory extension.

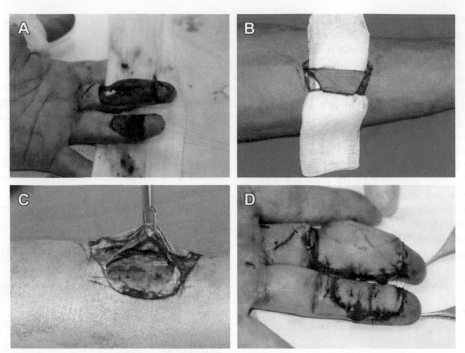

Fig. 13. Simultaneous reconstruction of neurovascular bundle and soft tissue defect. (*A*) Multiple digital soft tissue defect on volar side. Note 2 digital artery defect in each finger. (*B, C*) A venous free flap was raised from the ipsilateral forearm. (*D*) The flap veins were interposed as arterialized venous flap, which was followed by improved flow to the distal portion of the digits.

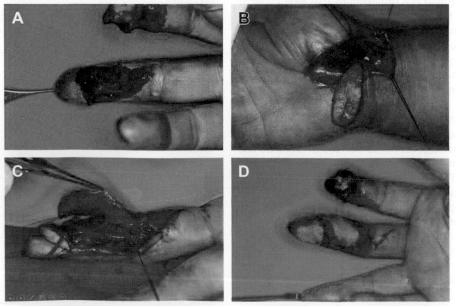

Fig. 14. Restoration of distal perfusion using a flow-through–type glabrous skin flap. (*A*) This long finger defect includes the loss of both digital arteries. Note the duskiness in the distal fingertip. (*B*) This thenar free flap was elevated with the artery in a flow-through configuration. (*C*) The flap is insetted with the vascular pedicle interposed between the proximal and distal ends of the digital artery. (*D*) In the immediate postoperative evaluation, the distal fingertip shows adequate circulation.

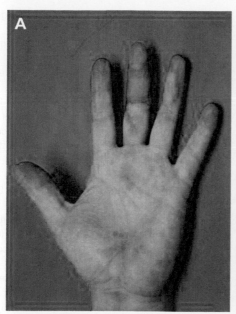 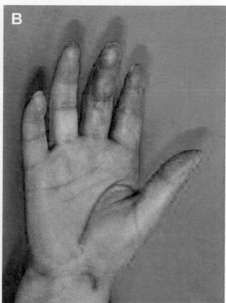

Fig. 15. Comparison between 2 flow-through–type free flaps. (*A*) At 9-month follow-up, venous free flap retains acceptable contour without contracture, but color and texture mismatch is noticeable. (*B*) At 6-month follow-up, the thenar free flap retains excellent color and texture matching.

difficult to reconstruct at the time of initial skin coverage operation. Extensor tendons do not have much excursion, however, and the tension can be controlled be tenodesis effect. As such, simultaneous reconstruction of extensor tendon and skin defect is a worthwhile consideration.[47] Vascularized tendocutaneous flap or tendofascial flap are reasonable 2-bird-1-stone solutions (**Fig. 11**). Multiple tendon reconstruction requires a delayed approach (**Fig. 12**).

Defects in neurovascular structures should be reconstructed at the time of initial operation, if at all possible.[48] Nerve or vessel segments can be harvested and grafted in isolation. In most cases of neurovascular injury, the easier solution is the venous free flap, using artery-to-artery interposition (**Fig. 13**). When possible, however, glabrous skin flap with a flow-through arterial pedicle is a superior option to restore the volar surface (**Fig. 14**). In the long term, venous flap is liable to develop volume atrophy, color change, and noticeable scar (**Fig. 15**).

Pedicled Flaps in Mutilated Hand Injuries

Although free flaps are increasingly used for soft tissue cover of the hand, there are instances where free tissue transfer is not technically possible or the required microsurgical skills are not available in the area.

The infraumbical part of the lower abdomen is well vascularized by superficial external iliac artery, superficial inferior epigastric artery, and the superficial external pudental artery. These vessels run from below upward and the para umbilical perforators radiating from the umbilicus. Although the perforator arteries have definite territories of supply, large areas of tissues are interconnected with vascular networks such that large flaps could be raised with a few, possibly single, perforator artery. Techniques have been refined in the usage of these flaps that good outcomes have been obtained by the use of these flaps.[49]

In addition, reverse flow flaps based on the radial artery and the posterior interosseous arteries have been used extensively for the provision of skin cover in the hand.[50–54] So present-day hand surgeons have a wide armamentarium to choose from when faced with the problem of provision of soft tissue cover in the hand so that good functional and aesthetic outcomes are achieved.

SUMMARY

The spectrum of free flaps discussed in this review represents the best practice options in mutilating hand injury for the following reasons:

1. Compared with local flaps, free flaps do not require additional morbidity at the injury site.
2. A single-stage reconstruction is possible even for multiple injuries.
3. Free flaps allow for maximal preservation of function.

4. A wide variety flap sizes and designs is available for free flaps.
5. Free flaps allow for restoration of normal contour.
6. Free flaps facilitate for functional reconstruction at the time of secondary operation (eg, provide a smooth surface for tendon reconstruction).[3]

Limitations of free flaps are the need for microsurgical technique, steep learning curve, and donor-site morbidity.

Because restoration of function is the primary goal of hand surgery, the most reliable reconstruction strategy for soft tissue defect seems to be the use of various free flaps. Among these, free fascial flap seems most suited for extensor surfaces, because it provides a thin, pliable interface with a smooth gliding surface. Because of the pliable characteristics, fascial free flaps are able to conform to the most complex configuration of wounds, which makes it all the more applicable to wounds resulting from mutilating injury. Although fascial flaps can be used for volar soft tissue defect in a pinch, glabrous skin flaps are more appropriate in most situations. This is especially important for distal volar tissue defects in digits.

The authors have emphasized the importance of considering various flaps for each component of a mutilating hand injury. Despite that free flap techniques have become widely popular in the past 2 decades, what remains true is that, for individual surgeons, free flaps still require a significant investment in training and personal time. Because of this, the choice of free flap is dictated not by clinical circumstance of an injury but by surgeon preference and training program. To abide by the principle of replacing like with like tissue, however, it is important that surgeons be comfortable in harvesting a wide variety of flaps to restore the shape and function to missing portions of a mutilated hand.

REFERENCES

1. Neumeister MW, Brown RE. Mutilating hand injuries: principles and management. Hand Clin 2003;19(1): 1–16.
2. del Piñal F. Severe mutilating injuries to the hand: guidelines for organizing the chaos. J Plast Reconstr Aesthet Surg 2007;60(7):816–27.
3. Jeon BJ, Yang JW, Roh SY, et al. Microsurgical reconstruction of soft-tissue defects in digits. Injury 2013;44(3):356–60.
4. Saint-Cyr M, Gupta A. Indications and selection of free flaps for soft tissue coverage of the upper extremity. Hand Clin 2007;23(1):37–48.
5. Engelhardt TO, Rieger UM, Schwabegger AH, et al. Functional resurfacing of the palm: flap selection based on defect analysis. Microsurgery 2012; 32(2):158–66.
6. Southwood WF. The thickness of the skin. Plast Reconstr Surg 1955;14:423–9.
7. Lee Y, Hwang K. Skin thickness of Korean adults. Surg Radiol Anat 2002;24(3–4):183–9.
8. Lutz BS, Wei FC, Chang SC, et al. Donor site morbidity after suprafascial elevation of the radial forearm flap: a prospective study in 95 consecutive cases. Plast Reconstr Surg 1999;103(1):132–7.
9. Hekner DD, Abbink JH, van Es RJ, et al. Donor-site morbidity of the radial forearm free flap versus the ulnar forearm free flap. Plast Reconstr Surg 2013; 132:387–93.
10. Lin TS, Jeng SF. Full-thickness skin graft as a one-stage debulking procedure after free flap reconstruction for the lower leg. Plast Reconstr Surg 2006;118(2):408–12.
11. Lin TS. One-stage debulking procedure after flap reconstruction for degloving injury of the hand. J Plast Reconstr Aesthet Surg 2016;69(5):646–51.
12. Hong JP, Choi DH, Suh H, et al. A new plane of elevation: the superficial fascial plane for perforator flap elevation. J Reconstr Microsurg 2014;30(7): 491–6.
13. Yousif NJ, Warren R, Matloub HS, et al. The lateral arm fascial free flap: its anatomy and use in reconstruction. Plast Reconstr Surg 1990;86:1138–45.
14. Chang SM. The distally based radial forearm fascia flap. Plast Reconstr Surg 1990;85:150–1.
15. Seradge H, Adham MN, Seradge E, et al. Free vascularized temporal parietal flap in hand surgery. Orthopedics 1995;18:1083–5.
16. Flügel A, Kehrer A, Heitmann C, et al. Coverage of soft-tissue defects of the hand with free fascial flaps. Microsurgery 2005;25(1):47–53.
17. Fassio E, Laulan J, Aboumoussa J, et al. Serratus anterior free fascial flap for dorsal hand coverage. Ann Plast Surg 1999;43:77–82.
18. Chen HC, el-Gammal TA. The lateral arm fascial free flap for resurfacing of the hand and fingers. Plast Reconstr Surg 1997;99:454–9.
19. Fox P, Endress R, Sen S, et al. Fascia-only anterolateral thigh flap for extremity reconstruction. Ann Plast Surg 2014;72(Suppl 1):S9–13.
20. Bhadkamkar MA, Wolfswinkel EM, Hatef DA, et al. The ultra-thin, fascia-only anterolateral thigh flap. J Reconstr Microsurg 2014;30(9):599–606.
21. Summers AN, Sanger JR, Matloub HS. Lateral arm fascial flap: microarterial anatomy and potential clinical applications. J Reconstr Microsurg 2000;16(4): 279–86.
22. Ki SH. Lateral arm free flap with preservation of the posterior antebrachial cutaneous nerve. Ann Plast Surg 2016;76(5):517–20.
23. Carty MJ, Taghinia A, Upton J. Fascial flap reconstruction of the hand: a single surgeon's

30-year experience. Plast Reconstr Surg 2010; 125(3):953–62.

24. Ninkovíc MM, Schwabegger AH, Wechselberger G, et al. Reconstruction of large palmar defects of the hand using free flaps. J Hand Surg Br 1997;22(5): 623–30.

25. Yoshimura M, Shimada T, Imura S, et al. The venous skin graft method for repairing skin defects of the fingers. Plast Reconstr Surg 1987;79:243–50.

26. Turner A, Ragowannsi R, Hanna J, et al. Microvascular soft tissue reconstruction of the digits. J Plast Reconstr Aesthet Surg 2006;59(5):441–50.

27. De Lorenzi F, van der Hulst RR, den Dunnen WF, et al. Arterialized venous free flaps for soft-tissue reconstruction of digits: a 40-case series. J Reconstr Microsurg 2002;18(7):569–74.

28. Kimata Y, Mukouda M, Mizuo H, et al. Second toe plantar flap for partial finger reconstruction. Plast Reconstr Surg 1998;101(1):101–6.

29. Cho YJ, Roh SY, Kim JS, et al. Second toe plantar free flap for volar tissue defects of the fingers. Arch Plast Surg 2013;40(3):226–31.

30. Kamei K, Ide Y, Kimura T. A new free thenar flap. Plast Reconstr Surg 1993;92:1380–4.

31. Omokawa S, Mizumoto S, Iwai M, et al. Innervated radial thenar flap for sensory reconstruction of fingers. J Hand Surg Am 1996;21(3):373–80.

32. Sassu P, Lin CH, Lin YT, et al. Fourteen cases of free thenar flap: a rare indication in digital reconstruction. Ann Plast Surg 2008;60(3):260–6.

33. Yang JW, Kim JS, Lee DC, et al. The radial artery superficial palmar branch flap: a modified free thenar flap with constant innervation. J Reconstr Microsurg 2010;26(8):529–38.

34. Shanahan RE, Gingrass RP. Medial plantar sensory flap for coverage of heel defects. Plast Reconstr Surg 1979;64(3):295–8.

35. Morrison WA, Crabb DM, O'Brien BM, et al. The instep of the foot as a fasciocutaneous island and as a free flap for heel defects. Plast Reconstr Surg 1983;72(1):56–65.

36. Sen SK, Fitzgerald O'Connor E, Tare M. The free instep flap for palmar and digital resurfacing. J Plast Reconstr Aesthet Surg 2015;68(9):1191–8.

37. Atasoy E, Ioakimidis E, Kasdan ML, et al. Reconstruction of the amputated finger tip with a triangular volar flap. A new surgical procedure. J Bone Joint Surg Am 1970;52(5):921–6.

38. Shepard GH. The use of lateral V-Y advancement flaps for fingertip reconstruction. J Hand Surg 1983;8:254–9.

39. O'Brien B. Neurovascular island pedicle flaps for terminal amputations and digital scars. Br J Plast Surg 1968;21:258–61.

40. Lee DC, Kim JS, Ki SH, et al. Partial second toe pulp free flap for fingertip reconstruction. Plast Reconstr Surg 2008;121(3):899–907.

41. Inoue T, Kobayashi M, Harashina T. Finger pulp reconstruction with a free sensory medial plantar flap. Br J Plast Surg 1988;41(6):657–9.

42. Huang SH, Wu SH, Lai CH, et al. Free medial plantar artery perforator flap for finger pulp reconstruction: report of a series of 10 cases. Microsurgery 2010; 30(2):118–24.

43. Kim KS, Kim ES, Hwang JH, et al. Fingertip reconstruction using the hypothenar perforator free flap. J Plast Reconstr Aesthet Surg 2013;66(9):1263–70.

44. Omokawa S, Ryu J, Tang JB, et al. Anatomical basis for a fasciocutaneous flap from the hypothenar eminence of the hand. Br J Plast Surg 1996;49(8): 559–63.

45. Kim HS, Lee DC, Kim JS, et al. Donor-Site Morbidity after Partial Second Toe Pulp Free Flap for Fingertip Reconstruction. Arch Plast Surg 2016;43(1):66–70.

46. Chim H, Ng ZY, Carlsen BT, et al. Soft tissue coverage of the upper extremity: an overview. Hand Clin 2014;30(4):459–73.

47. Yajima H, Inada Y, Shono M, et al. Radical forearm flap with vascularized tendons for hand reconstruction. Plast Reconstr Surg 1996;98(2):328–33.

48. Koshima I, Inagawa K, Sahara K, et al. Flow-through vascularized toe-joint transfer for reconstruction of segmental loss of an amputated finger. J Reconstr Microsurg 1998;14(7):453–7.

49. Sabapathy SR, Bajantri B. Indications, selection, and use of distant pedicled flap for upper limb reconstruction. Hand Clin 2014;30(2):185–99.

50. Higgins JP. A reassessment of the role of the radial forearm flap in upper extremity reconstruction. J Hand Surg Am 2011;36(7):1237–40.

51. Ho AM, Chang J. Radial artery perforator flap. J Hand Surg Am 2010;35(2):308–11.

52. Fong PL, Chew WY. Posterior interosseous artery flap: our experience and review of modifications done. Hand Surg 2014;19(2):181–7.

53. Acharya AM, Bhat AK, Bhaskaranand K. The reverse posterior interosseous artery flap: technical considerations in raising an easier and more reliable flap. J Hand Surg Am 2012;37(3):575–82.

54. Sabapathy SR, Bhardwaj P. Skin cover in hand injuries. Curr Orthop 2008;22(1):1–8.

Skeletal Fixation in a Mutilated Hand

Praveen Bhardwaj, MS (Ortho), DNB (Ortho), FNB (Hand & Microsurgery), EDHS,
Ajeesh Sankaran, MS (Ortho),
S. Raja Sabapathy, MS (Gen), MCh (Plastic), DNB (Plastic), FRCS (Edin), MAMS*

KEYWORDS

• Hand fracture • Mutilating injury • Wrist arthrodesis • Kirschner wire • Bone loss

KEY POINTS

- Hand fracture fixation in mutilating injuries is characterized by multiple challenges due to possible skeletal disorganization and concomitant severe injury of soft tissue structures.
- The effects of skeletal disruption are best analyzed as divided into specific locales in the hand: radial, ulnar, proximal, and distal. Functional consequences of injuries in each of these regions is discussed.
- Preventing contracture of the first web and extension contracture of the finger MCP joints is of paramount importance. Measures like prophylactic first web pinning, positioning during flap inset are elaborated.
- Given the myriad combinations of skeletal and soft tissue injuries possible, pointers like "make the hand look like a hand" or "more mutilation, more conservation" help simplify management.
- Although a variety of implants are now in vogue, K-wire fixation has stood the test of time and is especially useful in multiple fracture situations. Segmental bone loss is quite common in such injuries, which can be safely reconstructed in a staged manner.

Much of the intricate adaptability of the hand depends on the stable polyarticular skeleton being covered with pliable and sensate soft tissue. The goal of fracture fixation in severe injuries of the hand is to provide a backdrop stable enough for immediate reconstructive procedures. On the other hand, all soft tissue procedures must be planned with a view to achieve rapid and solid fracture healing in good position. Two factors that we have found detrimental to hand function in mutilating hand injuries are contracture of the first web and contracture of the metacarpal phalangeal (MCP) joints of the fingers. Their genesis lies less in the fracture pattern and more in the positioning after fixation. Planning only for fracture fixation gives a good radiograph, albeit of a nonfunctional hand. The goal is to achieve the best possible function under the circumstances. Setting course for such a defined goal should integrate the fixation plan with other procedures, such as flaps, nerve grafting, or tendon transfer. It is quite surprising how often the initial skeletal fixation turns out to be suboptimal for some future reconstruction. So, each milestone in the roadmap to salvage should be familiar to the entire team involved.

CHALLENGES IN FRACTURE FIXATION IN MUTILATED INJURIES

The mutilated hand differs from other closed injuries, or even most open fractures, in many ways. First, mutilating injuries may present with a disorganization of the skeleton. Before fracture fixation is considered, components that can be salvaged have to be identified.[1,2] These then need to be positioned for best possible function.

Second, mutilating injuries also present with joint disruption apart from the fractures. Restoring stability to these joints, while preserving motion, is

Department of Plastic, Hand & Reconstructive Microsurgery and Burns, Ganga Hospital, 313, Mettupalayam Road, Coimbatore, Tamil Nadu 641 043, India
* Corresponding author.
E-mail address: rajahand@gmail.com

Hand Clin 32 (2016) 505–517
http://dx.doi.org/10.1016/j.hcl.2016.06.001

hand.theclinics.com

quite a challenge. When ligaments and musculo-tendinous structures heal, it is very difficult to achieve the balance between pliability and strength they possess before injury. Bone healing, on the other hand, provides a wider latitude to restore normal function. Hence, a mutilated hand demands a determined effort to repair the soft tissues also along with the fractures, as early and as well as possible.

Third, the viability of a digit is influenced by the presence or absence of a fracture. We have observed that the prognosis of finger survival in degloving injuries is better when there are no phalangeal fractures. The addition of a fracture to this scene often results in a nonviable distal digit.

Finally, these fractures have a high incidence of nonunion or delayed union[3–5] as compared with closed or simple open fractures. Given the possibility of compromised hand function in these patients, a nonunion or delayed union is relatively more disabling and delays rehabilitation. In addition, access for secondary procedures for these nonunions is difficult due to precarious viability, scarring, and higher risk of neurovascular injury. For all the previously mentioned reasons, primary management of fractures in all major crush situations demands experience and patience.

EFFECTS OF SKELETAL DISRUPTION

Any fracture immediately introduces abnormal planes of movement to the adjacent soft tissues. When the soft tissues themselves are also significantly injured, the increased mobility compounds the insult. Partially injured vessels and nerves may suffer further injury if fractures are not splinted or fixed quickly enough. In addition, a fracture also represents injury of the attached muscle(s) and ligaments. The mobile tendinous units in the fingers undergo length changes in phalangeal fractures, with potential for eventual loss of motion of joints. Specific effects of skeletal injury in the hand are discussed as per specific regions: radial or ulnar and proximal or distal.

Radial Component

The thumb, index, and middle rays have been called the "dynamic tripod"[6] or the "dynamic tridactyl."[7] Precision grip capability is almost completely decided by the functional integrity of these rays. Injuries in which these are relatively spared or reliably reconstructed carry a better prognosis as regards eventual performance of fine activities. The most important problem to be addressed is the maintenance of the anteposed position of the thumb (**Fig. 1**). A thumb stiff in abduction is more useful than one stuck in adduction and extension.

Ulnar Component

The ring and little rays, along with the hypothenar eminence, are determinants of power grip activities by virtue of their more mobile metacarpals.[8]

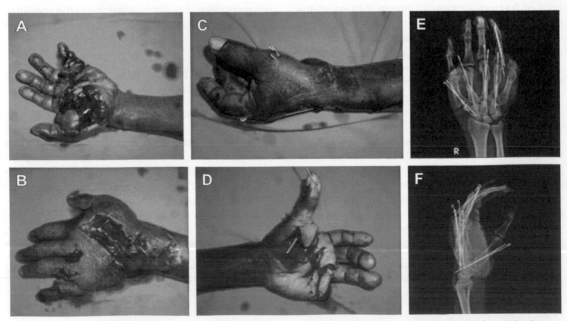

Fig. 1. (*A, B*) Preoperative clinical pictures of a press machine injury, with thenar wound. (*C, D*) After debridement and fracture fixation, demonstrating the abducted thumb. (*E, F*) Postoperative radiographs.

Skeletal fixation must be geared toward maintaining this strength and their position opposite to the thumb. Stiffness of one joint in these fingers can be compensated by the other joints to achieve good function, especially if the thumb is fully mobile. Conversely, nonunions and instability are poorly tolerated.

At least one radial and one ulnar component is the structural necessity of the "basic hand,"[9] that allows pinch. Positioning these rays to meet each other is the priority in fixation (**Fig. 2**). When more components are available or reconstructible, it is vitally important to position the thumb in a plane opposable to the rest. When a digit or ray is amputated, an intact radial ray may be translocated ulnarly to provide a wide span for grip and prevent first web contracture.[10] Loss of first web musculature cannot be modified by the surgeon and severely affects the result, as they contribute approximately 80% of the pinch strength.[11]

Proximal Component

The carpus and the metacarpals form the proximal skeletal component. Simply put, the wrist joint and the metacarpal "pillars" are involved in positioning the fingers around an object. In severe mutilations of this area, the ability to adapt the digits to a given object shape and consistency is hampered. Hence, the primary goal of fixation in these fractures is to provide a stable base for the salvaged fingers to move. With this view, primary wrist fusion may even be a good choice for complex injuries of the carpus or distal forearm (**Fig. 3**).

Distal Component

The phalanges are the adaptive mobile elements of the hand skeleton. Function of the fingers is determined mainly by the active movement range in the MCP and proximal interphalangeal (PIP) joints. Fixation in the fingers should allow early mobilization and avoid joint transfixion, except the distal interphalangeal (DIP) joint. The DIP may be primarily fused or the distal phalanx even sacrificed, to allow soft tissue cover.

PRIORITIES IN SKELETAL FIXATION
Make the Hand Look Like a Hand

Mutilating injuries present with a striking disorganization of the structure of the hand. The most grotesque of injuries can be salvaged with surprising amount of function, as long as this

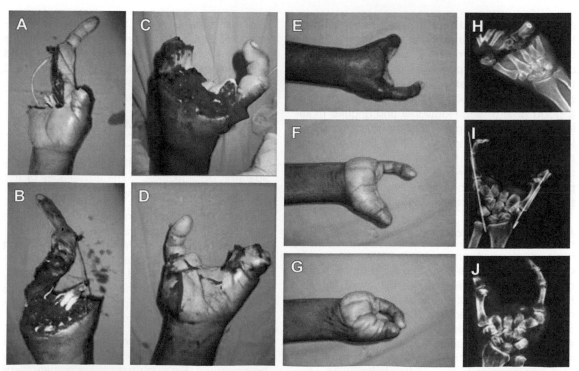

Fig. 2. (*A, B*) Severe mutilation of all rays, with only partially amputated thumb and avascular little finger available for reconstruction. (*C, D*) After revascularization of little finger and use of palmar skin to cover the thumb. The little ray has been fixed to ensure contact with the shortened thumb. (*E–G*) Postoperative function, with excellent pinch and span. No secondary reconstruction has been performed. (*H–J*) Preoperative, postoperative, and follow-up radiographs. Note the little finger has been stabilized to the ulna due to lack of carpal support.

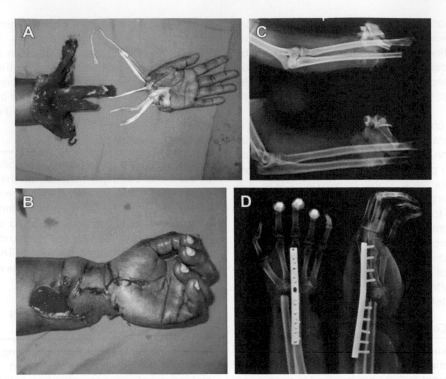

Fig. 3. Avulsion amputation at the carpus level preoperative and postoperative appearance (*A, B*). Preoperative and postoperative radiographs (*C, D*). Note the segmental fracture of radius, necessitating fusion to ulna.

structure is restored initially. The simple *mantra* to follow is "the hand should first look like a hand," as function follows form (**Fig. 4**). Severe comminution or bone loss often precludes proper reduction of fractures. In such situations, restoring alignment of the rays to correct the external appearance is a good goal to set. Rotational and angular malalignment has to be prevented, bone gaps may be left for later management. The fingers should achieve a cascade with the tips pointing toward the scaphoid tuberosity. The thumb should lie perpendicular to the palm. Any deviation from this is troublesome to manage at a later stage.

More the Mutilation, More the Conservation

In a single-digit crush injury, salvage may be considered doubtful if the expected function after reconstruction would hamper the other fingers.[3] However, when multiple digits are injured, salvage must be considered for each. A centimeter of saved length that allows a finger touch the thumb, considerably improves function of the entire hand.[12] Preserving the flexor digitorum superficialis (FDS) insertion to the middle phalanx with a flap rather than a proximal amputation provides PIP flexion and increases grip strength. A small retained segment of the base of the first metacarpal preserves the first carpometacarpal (CMC)

and dramatically widens the options for reconstruction (**Fig. 5**). An injured index finger that is considered nonsalvageable may actually be saved when translocated to replace an amputated thumb.[13] The fewer units available for salvage, the more each is worth the rescue.

Stabilize the Wrist and Mobilize the Fingers

A practical philosophy in complex injuries around the wrist region is to attain immediate stability by spanning plate fixation.[14] The advantages of this strategy being the following:

i. This stable background makes fixation and mobilization of distal fractures easier.
ii. The internal fixation offers no hindrance to soft tissue cover procedures.
iii. For many injuries, wrist fusion may be the only salvage possible and this may be performed as a definitive procedure primarily in major crush injuries with disorganized carpus.

In injuries in which the proximal forearm musculature is spared, pronosupination movements may be preserved. For such patients, a primary distal ulna resection along with the fusion allows this plane of motion to be salvaged (**Fig. 6**).

Primary arthrodesis is a reasonable option where carpal bones are crushed or lost, and

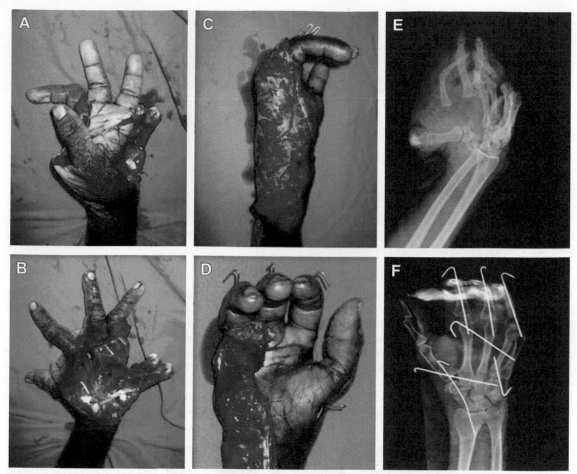

Fig. 4. (*A, B*) Disrupted architecture of the metacarpals. (*C, D*) "Making the hand look like a hand": functional position of joints achieved with fixation (free latissimus dorsi flap cover for ulnar defect). (*E, F*) Prefixation and postfixation radiographs.

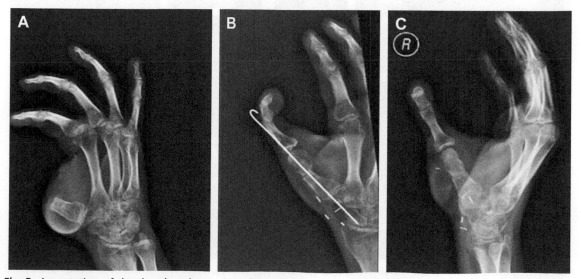

Fig. 5. Amputation of the thumb at base of the first metacarpal level (*A*). CMC joint has been salvaged with a pedicled abdominal flap, which allows good result with a second toe transfer (*B, C*).

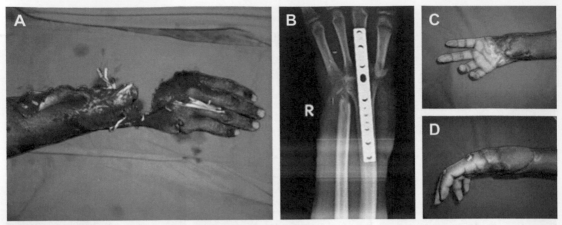

Fig. 6. Near total amputation at the carpus level (*A*) has been stabilized with a wrist fusion and distal ulna recession (*B*). This has preserved 90° of pronosupination arc (*C, D*).

favorable function has been reported.[15] Severe comminution of the radial articular surface is also an indication. When the radial articular cartilage is preserved, a proximal row carpectomy may be possible to restore wrist movement (**Fig. 7**).

Where fusion is not planned, the plate may be removed after 3 months when wounds have healed well. A minimal approach for implant removal is possible and should be used when no

other reconstructive procedure is planned in the same sitting.[14] It is important also to recognize at follow-up those patients who may need a secondary fusion. Whenever it is felt that restoring functional active movement of the wrist is not feasible, an arthrodesis should be a first choice and not considered an escape route. A painful wrist due to cartilage loss and a lack of motors are common indications for secondary fusion.

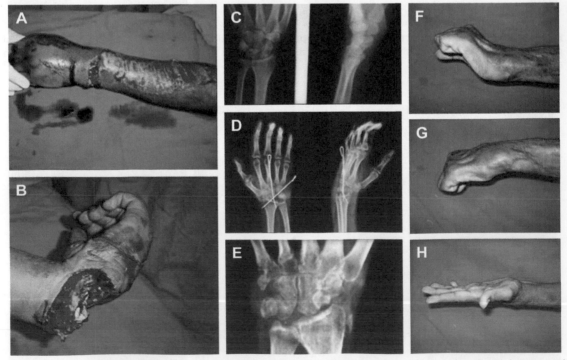

Fig. 7. Degloving injury of the dorsal hand and forearm (*A*), with cartilage loss of the ulnar head, lunate, and triquetrum (*B*). With the additional fracture of the scaphoid (*C*), a proximal row carpectomy was performed and stabilized with K-wires (*D*). The percutaneous wires allow early removal and mobilization, result at 15 months (*E–H*).

The wrist should be positioned in no more than 10° to 15° of extension for spanning fixation or fusion.[16] When finger extensors are weak, or expected to be so, the wrist should be fixed in neutral to allow some passive finger release. Also, a position of supination is preferable to pronation when temporary radioulnar stabilization is required, as the interosseous membrane is kept maximally stretched in partial supination. This position also allows easier inset of pedicled flaps from the abdominal region.

Focus on the First Web

Complete thumb amputation is the only condition more disabling than a severe first web contracture.[17] Thumb web contracture is a common sequel of mutilating hand injuries and needs to be kept in mind from the very beginning.[18] The flexor-adductor forces on the thumb are greater than the abductor forces that, along with gravity, produce a dynamic tendency for the first web to collapse.[19] Contracture could result from skin loss, contracture of the first web muscles, or just poor positioning of the thumb during the recovery phase. Ironically, the most easily preventable cause of contracture is also the commonest: improper positioning. The simple expedient of keeping the thumb maximally abducted at all times saves a lot of sweat later. In mutilating hand injuries, this positioning of the thumb is difficult, given the severity of the soft tissue injury and the position needed for flap inset. Nevertheless, all effort should focus on preventive measures right from the first procedure. It has been noted that even uninjured structures of the first web can progressively develop fibrosis,[20,21] thereby even a simple skin laceration has the potential for devastating contracture. Also, as the first webspace is a dynamic triangle with its apex at the bases of the metacarpals, injuries of this region can produce a great contraction of thumb-index span. Hence, if there are multiple skin wounds in the web area or fractures in proximity of the web apex, prophylactic fixation is warranted. An intermetacarpal Kirschner wire (K-wire) (**Fig. 8**) or an external fixator should be applied. First web contracture is also a disturbingly common sequel of an entire family of injuries involving direct pressure on the thenar area. They result in an avulsion of the first web muscles from their origins, left attached only at their insertions. These nonviable muscles get excised at debridement, leaving a dead space, paving the way for first web collapse. Such first web burst injuries also necessitate fixation to maintain the first web span. Blast injuries of the hand have also been noted to have a predilection for the radial rays

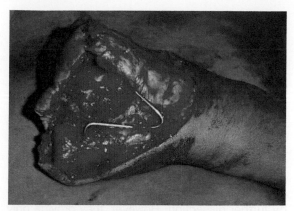

Fig. 8. Curved intermetacarpal wire to maintain the first web.

and first web involvement.[22,23] If there are no wounds over the web skin, a web spreader splint can maintain the space during the healing phase.

Keep the Metacarpophalangeal Joints Flexed

Flexion of the MCP joint is essential for hand function. All the basic grips of the hand, except the hook grip, need MCP flexion. Extension contracture is a common sequel of major hand injuries. Extended position of the MCP joints is the position of comfort because in this position the MCP joint cavity is most spacious. In an injured hand, edema is maximum over the dorsum and the stretched skin restricts flexion. The extensor tendons also displace dorsally, increasing their moment of action at the MCP joint. The MCP joint assumes an extended position where the collateral ligaments are lax.[24] If this position is not corrected, the ligaments fibrose and shorten, precluding flexion at the MCP joint. Once established, the extension contracture is exceedingly difficult to correct and most often will need an MCP capsulotomy with collateral ligament release. As in the case of the first web, the MCP contracture is also easier prevented than treated. Prevention of hand swelling by strict hand elevation and encouraging active finger movements is an effective measure. Careful fixation of the phalanx and metacarpal fractures with MCP held flexed is important. The K-wire entry point in the region of extensor apparatus is bound to cause problems by transfixion, so the MCP joints should be kept in flexion while passing the wires so as to prevent fixation of the MCP joint in extension. Anatomic differences predispose the fifth MCP to be the commonest to suffer in all contractures and is also always most severely involved.[25] In the early rehabilitation phase, a dorsal splint to block MCP extension and rubber hand traction to keep the MCP flexed is useful.

TECHNICAL ASPECTS
Implants

Kirschner wires

Wires or pins are the most common implants used in hand fracture fixation.[26–28] They are easily available, economical, and easy to apply, with a short learning curve. In major open injuries, K-wires can be quickly placed by retrograde wiring through the fracture site. This also prevents possible injury by further dissection. However, they provide only relative stability and generally do not facilitate immediate aggressive mobilization. A number of modifications have been described to improve construct rigidity.[29] Many of them involve extensive tissue dissection and/or involved placement of implants. We find crossed K-wires to be sufficient for most fractures, even in mutilating injuries. Although absolute stability may not be attained with any K-wiring technique, properly applied wire(s) have been known to be stable enough to achieve good outcomes. The commonly used wire sizes are 1.5 mm for the metacarpals and 1.25 mm or 1.1 mm for the phalanges.

Screws and plates

Lag screw fixation provides absolute stability and is well suited for long oblique/spiral fracture patterns.[29] Intra-articular exposure and intramedullary screw fixation for transverse fracture types has also been described and can be adapted to open fractures as well.[30] Multiple screw fixation also comes with the attendant complications of extensive devascularization of fragments for exposure. When possible, screws provide stable fixation with fewer hardware issues. So while they are of great value in simple fractures, screw fixation is hardly feasible for multiple fractures or in comminuted fractures (see **Fig. 1**).

Plate systems commonly used in the hand skeleton are "neutralization" or "bridging" constructs. Locking constructs are also becoming more popular.[31] They can be combined with lag screws to achieve compression, but do not per se provide absolute stability. Plating is expensive and somewhat technically demanding for inexperienced surgeons. Like screws, plates suffer from the same problems of wide soft tissue stripping and long time needed to fix multiple fractures. When they are used, screws seem more appropriate for phalangeal fractures and plates for metacarpal fractures[32]; 2.0-mm to 2.7-mm plates/screws are usually used for metacarpals, 1.5-mm to 2.0-mm for the proximal phalanges, and 1.3-mm to 1.5-mm ones for the middle phalanx.[33]

External fixators

A bewildering array of designs has been and continues to be described in the literature, from the simple to the complex.[34–39] They can be applied quickly and easily, even by a beginner. They also provide sufficient stability for early mobilization, while not requiring excessive devitalization. Hold of the fixator can be improved by using threaded pins[39]; however, some frames can be cumbersome and interfere with positioning of flaps. Malleable systems can also be used for multiple complex fracture situations, which incorporate some degree of dynamicity and potential for protected mobilization.[40]

The literature for implant selection in mutilating hand situations is quite sparse, so that no evidence-based recommendations can be made.[41] Plating systems have been shown to be biomechanically more stable constructs than others in both metacarpals[42] and phalanges[43]; however, hand fractures do not need to be united to begin mobilization.[27] K-wires are considered to provide enough stability for controlled mobilization.[27,44] Extensive soft tissue dissection and periosteal stripping with plating also increases hand edema, itself leading to stiffness.[45] Although complications are well known for plating systems,[45,46] K-wiring is also not without problems of contractures and infection.[47] In spite of the attractive theoretic advantage that construct stability provides in mutilating situations, some experts do prefer multiple K-wire fixation for being less time-consuming and when soft tissue viability is precarious.[48] Duncan and colleagues,[49] in their classic study of 75 open hand fractures, observed that grades I, II, and IIIA open fractures had 50% lesser final active range of motion when wounds were extended for fixation. As a general principle, they concluded that open hand fractures should be stabilized with the least invasive modality commensurate with biomechanical stability.

Specific Fractures

Phalanges

Distal phalanx Most such fractures, when they occur in mutilating injuries, are better left alone. Simple repair of the nailbed and pulp tissue suffices in hand mutilation scenarios. A single axial K-wire may be used when fixation is considered necessary. With severe comminution of the distal phalanx base or middle phalanx head, a single wire may be placed across the DIP joint to achieve fusion. In circumferential degloving injury of multiple fingers, the fingertips may need to be amputated at the DIP joint level to allow pedicled flap cover.

Middle phalanx The overriding principle in the management of these fractures is the preservation of the PIP joint ("the functional locus of finger function"[50]). Transfixing the PIP joint in extra-articular fractures is to be avoided, except when the central extensor slip is found injured. Displaced neck fractures may well be fixed with an axial wire across the DIP joint. Transverse shaft fractures are best served with crossed K-wires, although technically demanding given the narrow cross section of the bone involved. Additionally, the wires must be ensured to exit dead laterally. When the fingers are to be covered with a flap, the wires may be cut short and buried or be placed axially.

Proximal phalanx Straddled by both the MCP and PIP joints, the proximal phalanx deserves the greatest care in fixation. When these joints are involved in open injuries, prognosis for range of motion is poor. The only means available to the surgeon is early mobilization after stable fixation. Multiple wire fixation is the easiest and disturbs tissues the least. Keeping wires in the mid-lateral plane is the safest method to avoid transfixing the tendons, but could be impossible in multiplanar fractures. Screws are devoid of impingement problems and could be placed in compression mode for absolute stability. Screw fixation should be considered whenever they can be placed without any further exposure. Plates are best left for segmental comminution or bone gap situations.

Metacarpals
Second to fifth metacarpals As discussed previously, sparing the MCP joints and keeping them in a functional position is of prime importance. Reduction of neck or shaft fractures require the MCP joints to be kept in flexion. Wires also should be placed while holding full flexion and ensuring the extensors and the collateral ligaments are at their longest. With multiple wires, chances of transfixion of the extensor apparatus increase and greater care is needed. External fixators are quite handy for multiple metacarpal fracture situations. Plating is the other option, especially when comminution is severe or a pedicled flap for soft tissue cover is planned.

First metacarpal More than fracture reduction, it is the relative position of the first ray to the rest of the hand that is crucial. With soft tissue injury

in the first web, we prefer fixation with an intermetacarpal K-wire from the first to second metacarpal. The thumb should be placed in maximal abduction and in line with the radial border of the index finger, with enough pronation so that the pulp points to the pulps of other fingers. The wire is driven as distally as possible at the base of the first web triangle. This prevents further injury to the first web muscles. When skin and muscle loss is present, a triangle or quadrilateral frame external fixator is a better choice.[18]

SEGMENTAL BONE LOSS

Littler[51] has suggested that the metacarpals and phalanges are in a definite length ratio to one another. Loss of length in even any one component can compromise the motion arc and may affect function in ways yet unfathomed.

Bone loss of the distal phalanx is usually managed by shortening the fingertip. Balancing the pulp and nailbed tissues to the proportion of distal phalanx available gives a normal contour of the tip with proper nail growth. If required, a peg bone graft can be packed under the nailbed.[52]

Bone loss in the middle and proximal phalanges produces the most unsightly deformities, with loss of function. At the initial stabilization, the correct length of these bones is maintained by various techniques. This length is determined by comparison with the segments of the adjacent fingers. When multiple fingers are injured, proper length can be achieved only by placing the soft tissues optimally. Overstretching the tissues can precipitate vascular insufficiency and must be avoided. Spacer wires or external fixators are commonly used to maintain length temporarily in the face of bone loss.[53] Defects spanning articular areas can be temporarily or definitively filled by a silicone spacer.[54] Fixators can be retained after the definitive bone grafting until union; however, they are unwieldy when multiple bone segments are involved. Spanning plate fixation works on a similar "internal fixator" principle and can be converted to definitive fixation as well.

Acute management of metacarpal bone loss is quite similar. Multiple adjacent metacarpals are more likely to be involved than the phalanges. Proper length is achieved by assessing the knuckle prominence. Normally the middle metacarpal is distalmost, at the apex of a smooth distal convex arc.

The timing of the definitive grafting is crucial. Complete loss of the graft due to infection or an

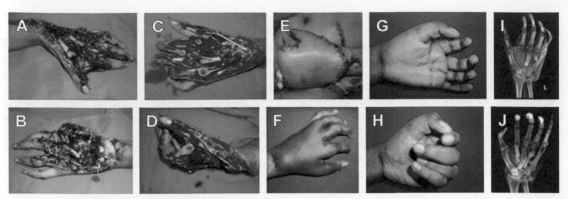

Fig. 9. (*A, B*) Severe dorsal mutilation with soft tissue and bone loss. (*C, D*) After debridement and stabilization to maintain hand joints in functional position. (*E*) Pedicled groin flap cover, maintaining the thumb abduction and MCP flexion. (*F–H*) Postoperative clinical result. (*I, J*) Radiographs before and after bone grafting.

avascular bed is quite possible, while restored length decreases infection and edema by eliminating dead space.[55] Single-stage combined soft tissue and bony reconstruction is often cited, with improved outcomes.[55–57] In our practice, we prefer staged reconstruction for wounds with precarious margins. Soft tissue cover is achieved first. Bone grafting is done when the induration and edema of the flap settles (**Fig. 9**). However, in a clean wound with doubtless viable margins, the flap and bone grafting are combined (**Fig. 10**).[58]

Various types of graft donor areas and methods have been described over the years.[59–64] Most defects in salvageable injuries are lesser than 6 cm, small enough for nonvascularized grafts. We are unsure of the value of the vascularized graft in hand mutilation and have not had occasion to use it. Small defects in the phalanges are best filled by a corticocancellous iliac crest chunk. Larger defects are served better by a

cortical strut. While grafting for phalanges, care must be taken to avoid overstuffing the graft. This is in itself a cause of stiffness and also risks wound breakdown.

Multiple metacarpal defects can be managed with a large composite block iliac crest graft,[59] especially those of the less mobile second and third metacarpals. Separate grafting of each metacarpal theoretically allows more motion, but its clinical effect on function may be minimal. Leaving the fifth metacarpal out of a composite graft for independent function antipodal to the first ray should be enough.

The "induced membrane" technique by Masquelet[65] has been described for bone loss in the hand as well. Although this is a promising technique, the staged nature of the graft may compound stiffness due to the time taken to achieve skeletal stability.[66] Thermal injury to the neurovascular bundles of the finger by the heat of cementing is also a risk.

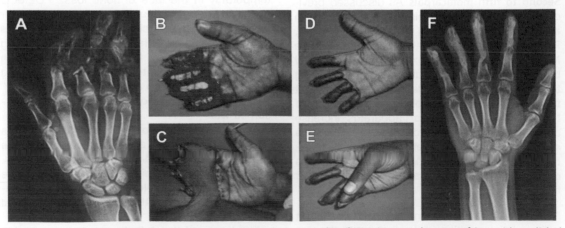

Fig. 10. (*A*) Bone loss of all fingers distal to proximal phalanx. (*B, C*) Single-stage bone grafting with pedicled groin flap cover. (*D, E*) Postoperative clinical result. (*F*) Postoperative radiograph after graft take.

SUMMARY

Skeletal fixation of mutilating hand injuries should be geared toward 3 basic goals: preservation of structure, restoration of motion, and prevention of deformities. No two injuries are the same and, hence, no formula for fracture fixation can be drawn up. Given the variety of options for fixation now available, the final choice should be based on the resources and expertise accessible. Rather than the method chosen, it is the strict adherence to basic principles that often decides the outcome of such injuries.

REFERENCES

1. Arellano AO, Wegener EE, Freeland AE. Mutilating injuries to the hand: early amputation or repair and reconstruction. Orthopedics 1999;22(7):683–4.

2. Tos P, Artiaco S, Titolo P, et al. Limits of reconstruction in mangled hands. Chir Main 2010;29(4):280–2.

3. Ring D. Malunion and nonunion of the metacarpals and phalanges. Instr Course Lect 2006;55:121–8.

4. Chow SP, Pun WK, So YC, et al. A prospective study of 245 open digital fractures of the hand. J Hand Surg 1991;16(2):137–40.

5. Swanson TV, Szabo RM, Anderson DD. Open hand fractures: prognosis and classification. J Hand Surg 1991;16(1):101–7.

6. Capener N. The hand in surgery. J Bone Joint Surg Br 1956;38B(1):128–51.

7. Tubiana R, Thomine JM, Mackin E. Examination of the hand and wrist. 2nd edition. London: Martin Dunitz; 1998.

8. Napier JR. The prehensile movements of the human hand. J Bone Joint Surg Br 1956;38B(4):902–13.

9. Burkhalter W. Mutilating injuries of the hand. In: Hunter JM, Mackin EJ, Callahan AD, editors. Rehabilitation of the hand: surgery and therapy. St Louis (MO): Mosby; 1995. p. 1037–56.

10. Elliot D, Henley M, Sammut D. Selective replantations with ulnar translocation in multidigital amputations. Br J Plast Surg 1994;47(5):318–23.

11. Hastings H 2nd, Davidson S. Tendon transfers for ulnar nerve palsy. Evaluation of results and practical treatment considerations. Hand Clin 1988;4(2):167–78.

12. Mathew P, Venkatramani H, Sabapathy SR. Mini-abdominal flaps for preservation of digital length in an 18-month old child. J Hand Surg Eur 2013;38(1):89–91.

13. Raja Sabapathy S, Sebastin SJ, Venkatramani H, et al. Primary use of the index finger for reconstruction of amputated thumbs. Br J Plast Surg 2004;57(1):50–60.

14. Vedder NB, Hanel DP. The mangled upper extremity. In: Wolfe SW, Hotchkiss RN, Pederson WC, et al, editors. Green's operative hand surgery. 6th edition. Philadelphia: Churchill Livingstone; 2011. p. 1603–44.

15. De la Rosa- Massieu D, Gonzales- Sanchez M, Onishi Sadud W, et al. Severe hand injury due to a high energy gunshot projectile treated with arthrodesis of the carpus, synthetic bone graft and external fixators. Case report. Acta Ortop Mex 2014;28(4):240–3.

16. Bhardwaj P, Nayak SS, Kiswar AM, et al. Effect of static wrist position on grip strength. Indian J Plast Surg 2011;44(1):55–8.

17. Jobe MT. Compartment syndromes and Volkmann contracture. In: Canale ST, editor. Campbell's operative orthopedics. 9th edition. St Louis (MO): Mosby; 1998. p. 3661–71.

18. Del Pinal F, Garcia-Bernal FJ, Delgado J. Is post-traumatic first web contracture avoidable? Prophylactic guidelines and treatment oriented guidelines. Plast Reconstr Surg 2004;113(6):1855–60.

19. Brand PW, Hollister AM. Mechanics of individual muscles at individual joints. In: Brand PW, Hollister AM, editors. Clinical mechanics of the hand. 3rd edition. St Louis (MO): Mosby; 1999. p. 100–83.

20. Herrick RT, Lister GD. Control of first webspace contracture. Including a review of the literature and tabulation of opponensplasty techniques. Hand 1977;9(3):253–64.

21. Sandzen SC Jr. Thumb web reconstruction. Clin Orthop Relat Res 1985;(15):66–82.

22. Hazani R, Buntic RF, Brooks D. Patterns in blast injuries to the hand. Hand (N Y) 2009;4(1):44–9.

23. Adhikari S, Bandyopadhyay T, Sarkar T, et al. Blast injuries to the hand: pathomechanics, patterns and treatment. J Emerg Trauma Shock 2013;6(1):29–36.

24. Smith P. Lister's the hand: diagnosis and indications. 4th edition. London: Churchill Livingstone; 2002.

25. Simpson RL, Flaherty ME. The burned small finger. Clin Plast Surg 1992;19(3):673–82.

26. Gregory S, Lalonde DH, Fung Leung LT. Minimally invasive finger fracture management: wide-awake closed reduction, K-wire fixation, and early protected movement. Hand Clin 2014;30(1):7–15.

27. Henry MH. Fractures of the proximal phalanx and metacarpals in the hand: preferred methods of stabilization. J Am Acad Orthop Surg 2008;16(10):586–95.

28. Palibrk TD, Lesić AR, Andjelković SZ, et al. Operative treatment of metacarpal and phalangeal fractures with Kirschner wire fixation–a review. Acta Chir Iugosl 2013;60(2):49–52.

29. Day CS, Stern PJ. Fractures of the metacarpals and phalanges. In: Wolfe SW, Hotchkiss RN, Pederson WC, et al, editors. Green's operative hand surgery. 6th edition. Philadelphia: Churchill Livingstone; 2011. p. 239–90.

Primary Thumb Reconstruction in a Mutilated Hand

Francisco del Piñal, MD, Dr Med[a,b,*],
Davide Pennazzato, MD[c], Esteban Urrutia, MD[d]

KEYWORDS

- Ectopic replantation • Toe-to-hand transfer • Partial thumb defects • Mutilating injuries

KEY POINTS

- Thumb reconstruction is the priority in any reconstructive plan.
- Toe transfer is an effective method of thumb reconstruction.
- Trim toe transfer (from great toe) gives better result than second toe transfer.
- Reducing the donor site morbidity by transfer of second toe to the harvested great toe site increases patient satisfaction and acceptance of the procedure.
- Conventional techniques like pollicization and Littler neurovascular island flap can be helpful in patients who decline toe transfer or do not have toes.

INTRODUCTION

Without doubt, the most effective way of restoring the amputated thumb function is by replanting it. Any major effort is justifiable to do so. This article discusses succinctly the classic alternatives and expends more time on others. **Box 1** summarizes the ideal methods (the first being replantation, not discussed here) and contains the topics dealt with in this article.

Ectopic Banking

Ectopic banking was first described by Marco Godina.[1] It consists of temporarily reconnecting an amputated or devascularized element in a nonanatomic position. The main reasons for doing so are in cases where there is concomitant major soft tissue damage around the thumb or if the patient is critically ill, and thus major surgery is not wise. The rationale to indicate ectopic banking in the former case is that debridement can be staged, and cover can be delayed, while in the latter, surgery can be carried out expeditiously and under regional anesthesia. Most authors have found the ideal place for ectopic replantation as the contralateral forearm.[2] Generally, after several weeks, the digit is elevated in continuity with the radial artery and local veins, thus preserving the previous anastomoses, and planted in the proper location. In most published cases, a flap in continuity, or a flap from another location, is needed concomitantly. This is so, because as stated previously, the major indication for ectopic replantation is precisely an associated soft tissue defect.

The authors must confess that their personal experience with ectopic banking of digits is nil. This is so, because although there is an indication for resorting to ectopic replantation in the fatidic

[a] Instituto de Cirugía Plástica y de la Mano, Hospital La Luz, Madrid, Spain; [b] Instituto de Cirugía Plástica y de la Mano, Hospital Mutua Montañesa, Santander, Spain; [c] Orthopaedics and Traumatology, Department of Biotechnology and Life Sciences (DBSV), University of Insubria, Varese, Italy; [d] Department of Orthopaedic Surgery, School of Medicine, Pontificia Universidad Catolica de Chile, Santiago, Chile
* Corresponding author. Calle de Serrano 58-1B, Madrid E-28001, Spain.
E-mail addresses: drpinal@drpinal.com; pacopinal@gmail.com

Hand Clin 32 (2016) 519–531
http://dx.doi.org/10.1016/j.hcl.2016.07.004
0749-0712/16/© 2016 Elsevier Inc. All rights reserved.

coincidence of a major soft tissue defect around the amputated thumb and a critically ill patient, the authors believe most other cases can be solved by means of combining a (flow-through) free flap at the same time as the replantation. Despite the fact that at first glance it may be considered as a nonsensical venture, thinking objectively, it is not. The flap permits one to skip the area of damage in the thumb and proximal stump, allowing much faster and safer anastomoses, as the surgeon can much more radically debride damaged tissues. The authors' preferred flap is the dorsalis pedis (**Fig. 1**), but the contralateral radial forearm flap (perhaps the only indication the authors have found for using this flap presently) is even better.

Lesser catastrophic soft tissue losses can be dealt by local flaps. For dorsal defects, the authors

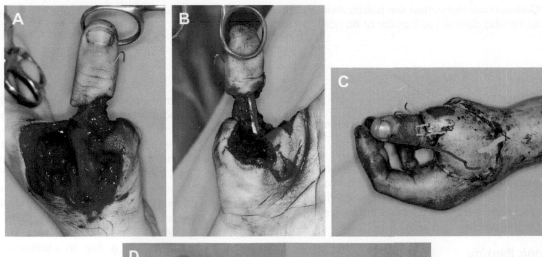

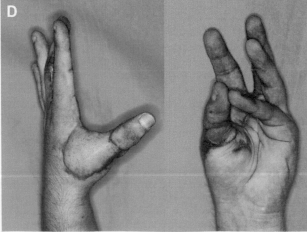

Fig. 1. (*A*) Status after debridement and fixation of the thumb in its position demonstrating massive soft tissue defect. (*B*) The dorsalis pedis flap has been used as an arterial and vein carrier. (*C*) Function 8 weeks after the accident. (*D*) Result. (Copyright © 2016 Dr Piñal.)

will underscore the utility of the first dorsal metacarpal flap as their preferred flap (**Fig. 2**).[3] Not only will this flap permit closure of moderate size defects, but it can be used as a vein carrier, avoiding the use of interpositional veins. For palmar defects, the authors would opt for an island flap from the ulnar aspect of the index or radial aspect of the middle[4] and transpose it to the volar aspect of the thumb. Not only will this provide cover, but also healthy arterial inflow.

Ectopic Replantation (Spare Parts Replantation)

Ectopic replantation consists of replanting a part away from its anatomic position. In the case here presented to replant an amputated finger onto the thumb position.

The authors' own results with ectopic replantation have not been as satisfactory as other authors might have found. The thumb that one obtains after such an operation is much less sturdy and thin, providing a poor surface for opposition. This is partly because any finger is thinner than the thumb, and because fat atrophy after replantation always occurs. Nevertheless, ectopic replantation has the unarguable advantage of not requiring sacrificing a toe. It should be stressed that a stiff index finger with poor sensibility will be skipped

during pinch. For this reason, the best indication for ectopic replantation is an amputated index finger proximal to the proximal interphalangeal (PIP) joint, and a nonreplantable thumb. The technique of ectopic replantation is exactly the same as standard replantation, except that the structures will not match. The surgeon has to be prepared to sort this problem out by using interpositional vein grafts as required, particularly for the veins (**Fig. 3**).

Major Intercalated Defects

A painful, insensate, or unstable thumb is, functionally speaking, as much use as having no thumb at all; the patient would not use it. So, despite the fact that it may look less dramatic than when a thumb is lost, the wary surgeon should try to use all resources when dealing with such scenarios.

Major defects of bone/nerve/soft tissue are managed in the authors' practice resorting to the toe, and in most circumstances to the second toe (**Fig. 4**).[5–8]

- Despite the modifications needed according to the contents of the flap, the technique of elevation is similar to all partial toe flaps. All dissection is carried out with 3.5× loupes, and the leg is exsanguinated by elevation. This is so, because it is crucial when dissecting the veins

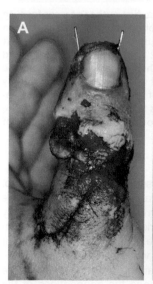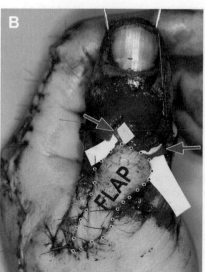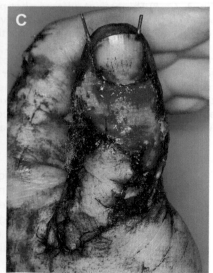

Fig. 2. (*A*) This patient was referred 48 hours after replantation for impending venous failure. The thumb drainage seemed to be strangled by the shortage of soft tissues, and the previous surgeons already used a local flap in attempt to overcome this, actually compounding the problem. (*B*) A 1.0 × 2.5 cm first dorsal metacarpal flap has been elevated from the dorsum of the index, permitting primary closure of the donor site. The flap eased the circular soft tissue constriction of the thumb, and most importantly carried 2 veins that reestablished the amputated part drainage (*blue arrows*). (*C*) Complete survival at 2 weeks. (Copyright © 2016 Dr Piñal.)

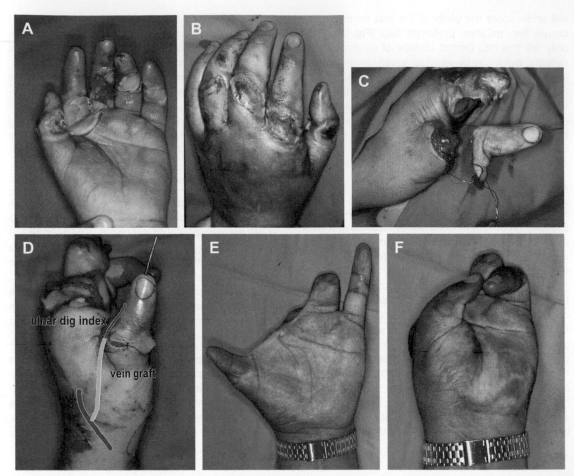

Fig. 3. (*A, B*) This patient suffered a hot-press injury 23 years ago (too early on in the first author's career for such a complex case). The fingers were unsalvageable, and only the index could be replanted in the thumb position (*C*). Primary arterial anastomoses to the thumb digital arteries provided only sluggish flow. (*D*) A long vein graft to the radial artery solved the problem. (*E, F*) The result is shown at 1 year. Note: a much better option would have been to replant the index distal to the PIP joint on the middle finger and then to carry out a second toe transfer to the stump of the ring finger and a hallux to the thumb. This patient was unwilling to pursue any reconstruction, perhaps influenced by the surgeon's hesitant attitude at the time of proposing the operation. Patients need to have a clear plan and a strong conviction by the surgeon that that is the best option. If not, in the authors' experience, they would reject reconstruction 9 times out of 10. See **Fig. 9** for the current management of a similar case. (Copyright © 2016 Dr Piñal.)

that they contain some blood for identification. Vein harvesting is sometimes the most difficult part of the whole operation, as veins are very small, and might be easily damaged. The authors used to do the dissection of the veins going from the distal edge of the flap and then directed proximally. This is very time consuming, and the tiny veins are at risk. Now the authors prefer to dissect the veins in the dorsum of the foot and track the vein and its branches distally, to the proximal edge of the flap. This is much faster and safer. Contrarily, the digital artery is located distally and traced proximally. Usually the digital artery is the donor

artery, and the dissection stops at the toe web. Once the vessels are isolated, elevation of the flap itself is carried out expeditiously, by following the periosteum and flexor sheath plane with a knife. The nerve is included or not depending on whether it is needed.

- In the osseous variant, great care should be taken not to damage the connections of the soft tissue to the bone and the vessels. The bone type flap also adds some extra difficulties at the time of elevating the bone from the opposite side of the pedicle. The digital artery of the other side would remain as the only source of blood supply to the toe. Staying

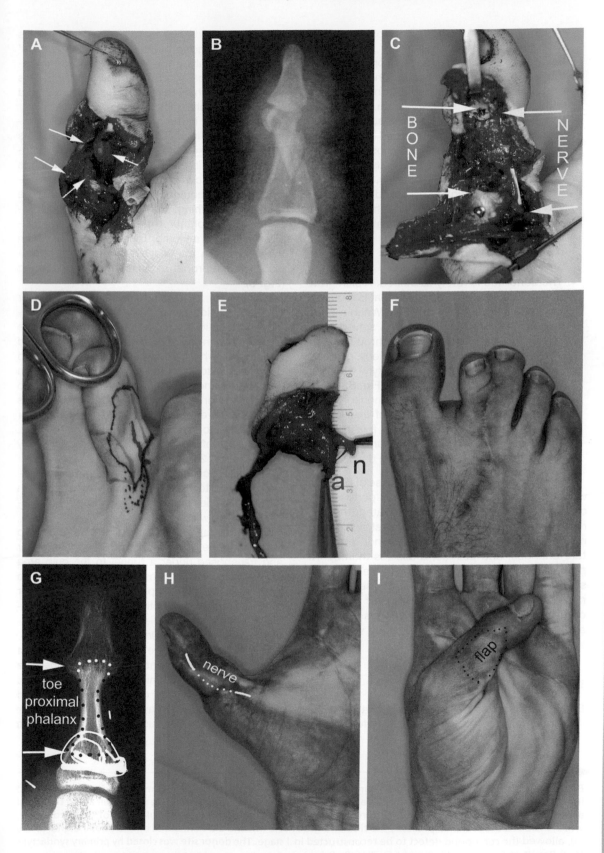

close to the periosteum of the phalanx, one will safeguard the artery.

- Once the flap is fitted into position, the anastomoses are carried out. The authors' preferred suture technique is running suture with 10/0 nylon in a 100 μ needle for both artery and vein. Two or three epineural stitches with the same material are placed in the nerve.
- After completion of the anastomoses and just before tourniquet release, a bolus of 1500 U heparin is injected intravenously. Thereafter, a continuous infusion of heparin diluted in saline at a rate of 250 to 500 U per hour is given for 4 days, which is reduced by half on the fifth day. Patients are discharged on day, 6 receiving low molecular weight heparin for an average of 2 more weeks.
- The donor toe is rarely sacrificed. A skin graft applied to the periosteum is all that is required in the soft tissue variants flaps. When a phalanx is harvested, usually this is solved by a resection arthroplasty or arthrodesis. In some cases in which a large piece of bone has been harvested, a syndactyly with the third toe is carried out (see also **Fig. 8**).
- Postoperatively, the flaps are monitored by the help of Doppler and color of the flap by the nurse on an hourly basis for the first 48 hours, thereafter every 2 hours except at nights (every 3 hours) for 2 more days.

The authors have also faced the case of patients whose thumb is alive but marginally perfused by dorsal arterial branches. If left untreated, the end result is a shrunken thumb with dystrophic nail, minimal sensibility, intolerance to minor temperature changes, and pain (ie, a useless thumb). To prevent this scenario, or to treat it in the subacute setting, flow-through versions of the second toe neurocutaneous flap are unparalleled.[9] This type of flap provides good cover (always needed), and, at the same time, pristine quality vessels to skip small defects (**Fig. 5**).

TERMINAL DEFECTS

Box 2 summarizes the methods available in the literature to reconstruct terminal defects. The authors must advance that the discussion of this subheading is going to be biased. In the authors' hands, the results a toe transfer gives to the patient are unsurpassed by any other method. This restricts the authors to rarely or never recommend some of the techniques available.

For example, in the authors' practice, it is difficult to find an indication for operations such as the Gillies cocked-hat, or the Matev first metacarpal lengthening. These time-honored methods are out of the current dot-com world in the authors' view. Although a bone lengthening may be better than nothing, the procedure at best procures a very poor thumb: no nail, no pulp, and usually too short of a thumb. These patients for whom those solutions may have served, totally appreciate when a proper reconstruction is performed (**Fig. 6**).

Conversely, other alternatives (eg, the Littler flap, pollicization of an index finger and, particularly, pollicization of a useless stump) might have a role in the armamentarium. The first is reserved for patients who have an exposed skeleton and do not want a toe transfer at any price. Pollicization is for the same group of patients who have no bone framework to cover. Pollicization of a useless stump, however, can be a definitive operation or might serve to reduce the needs from the foot. The authors often use this last option, and very rarely the first 2 options.

These 3 procedures are based on the same principle: to skeletonize the part to be transplanted in the volar arteries and nerves and move it as an island to the new location.

The Littler flap[10] consists of a neurovascular flap taken from the ulnar aspect of the middle finger and transposed under a tunnel to the pulp area of the thumb, thus providing sensibility to the pulp. Classically, the flap was the last stage after a neo-thumb reconstruction with a tube flap, usually an osteocutaneous flap from the groin, to provide sensibility to the palmar aspect of the thumb. According to Littler, there was no need to connect any nerve, as the patient will learn to reorientate the sensibility from the middle finger to the thumb. The authors, as several others have, have found that patients actually may be permanently disoriented, and might not use the thumb due to this

Fig. 4. (*A, B*) This 19-year-old patient sustained a crush to his left thumb. (*C*) Apart from the obvious bony loss and interphalangeal joint destruction, the radial digital nerve and a soft tissue cover were missing all along the radial aspect of the thumb. (*D–F*) An osteo-neuro-cutaneous flap harvested from the fibular side of the second toe, which included the proximal phalanx, the fibular digital nerve (n), and the skin, based on the fibular digital artery (a), allowed the compound defect to be reconstructed in 1 stage. The donor site was closed by primary syndactyly. (*G–I*) Result at 6 months. (Copyright © 2016 Dr Piñal.)

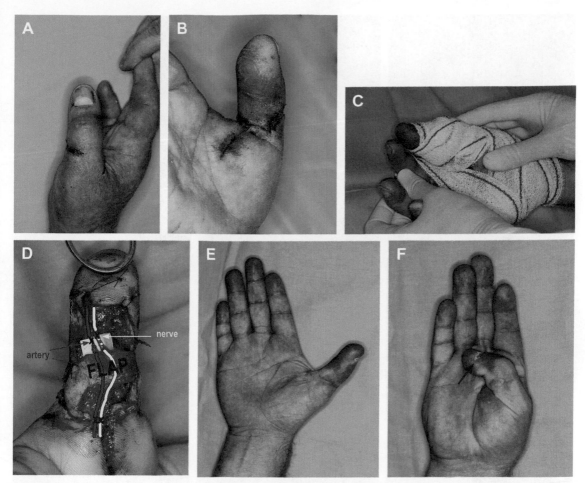

Fig. 5. (*A*) This patient was referred 3 weeks after his injury with an insensate and hypovascularized thumb after having sustained a near-circular injury. No Doppler sign could be detected. The marginal blood supply can be inferred by the bluish discoloration of the nail bed (*B*) and is much more evident at the time of surgery when the tourniquet was released (*C*). (*D*) A second toe neurovascular flap restored the arterial inflow as well as the ulnar digital nerve. (*E*, *F*) A useful painless thumb was obtained, but the damage at the nail matrix during the ischemic period produced a dystrophic nail (*arrow*). (Copyright © 2016 Dr Piñal.)

Box 2
Classic thumb reconstruction methods

- Cock-up of Gillies
- Matev metacarpal lengthening
- Littler type operations
  - ○ **Neurovascular flap**
  - ○ Pollicization
  - ○ **Stump transplantation**
- **Toe-to-hand transfer**

The authors preferred methods are in bold.

---

lack of proper sensibility. For this reason, provided there are nerves available, it is wiser to perform a neurorrhaphy between the recipient thumb nerves and the donor middle nerve to avoid cortical disorientation. As mentioned previously, the authors find this flap indicated for the patient who has some bone exposed and who does not want to have a more complex reconstruction (**Fig. 7**).

Pollicization consists of moving the index to the thumb position. Again, the authors must say from the beginning, that conceptually, except in severe forms of thumb hypoplasia, they rarely find room to recommend this operation. In adults, transposing an index results in a much thinner thumb

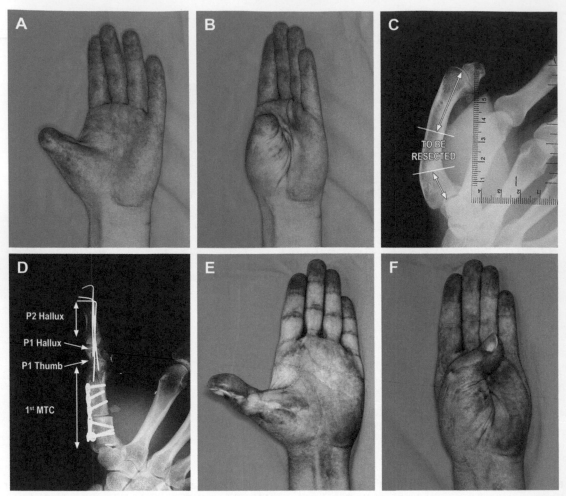

Fig. 6. (*A, B*) This 35-year-old sustained at the age of 20 a traumatic thumb amputation that was managed by lengthening. He had been seeking a better alternative ever since. (*C, D*) The author offered to straighten and shorten the metacarpal, and at the same time to carry out a trimmed toe hallux transfer. (*E, F*) Result at 3 years. (Copyright © 2016 Dr Piñal.)

than the original, and, worst of all, one sacrifices a finger.[11] Needless to say, in a severely mutilated hand, the indication of transposing a finger is nearly zero in the authors' view, as this will decrease the functional potential of the mutilated hand even further.

Nevertheless, a useless radial stump may be extremely useful for lengthening a short thumb and to increase the first web. Also, a radial stump may serve to decrease the needs from the foot. Apart from these, there are 2 more indications that the authors can foresee: the patient who does not want a toe transfer, or the patient who does not have a toe available for transfer (**Fig. 8**).

Technically speaking, these procedures (Littler, pollicization or stump transfer) are quite similar and based on the same principle. The flaps are

designed so the neothumb fits in its new place with the correct orientation. The neurovascular bundles are dissected as conservatively as possible (see **Fig. 7**C). If there are doubts about the integrity of the radial bundle and if the neighbor finger is correctly vascularized by the opposite side, the common digital artery of the ulnar side of the transferred segment is also included with the portion to be transplanted. Although for a Littler-type flap the venae comitans that accompany the digital artery are sufficient to allow safe venous drainage, in the case of a major segment, a dorsal vein needs to be included. As a rule, the nerves are minimally dissected and reconnected to the proximal stumps of the thumb digital nerves. Only in the event that the nerves have been avulsed proximally, is this step omitted.

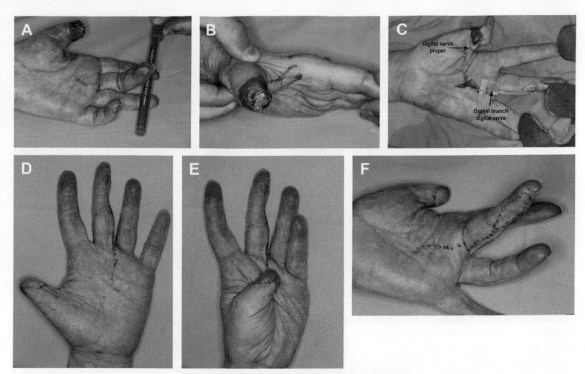

Fig. 7. (*A, B*) This 68-year-old patient suffered an avulsion amputation of her thumb with the seat belt as well as thoracic trauma in a car accident 10 days prior to her visit. She rejected a toe transfer, but accepted reconstruction with local tissues. To keep all the remaining bone, a large Littler flap, which allowed coverage of the palmar and dorsal defect, was planned. In order to increase the effective length of the thumb, a double opposing Z-plasty was done concomitantly. (*C*) The flap has now been elevated and prepared to be transposed under a skin tunnel. Notice that the dorsal branch of the donor nerve has been kept in place (*arrow*) and that only the palmar nerve proper has been harvested and is prepared for suturing to the ulnar digital nerve of the thumb (*arrow*). (*D, E*) The function at 1 year is shown. (*F*) The donor site was partially closed and the remaining defect covered with a full-thickness skin graft. (Copyright © 2016 Dr Piñal.)

Toe-to-Hand Transfer

When a patient has lost a thumb, the best option is a toe-to-hand transfer. The authors have found that even compensated amputations (distal to the IP joint) benefit enormously from toe transfer.[12] Nevertheless, the benefits of adding a toe, rather than removing anything from a mutilated hand, are self-evident.

The authors' preferred method for thumb reconstruction is by tailoring the hallux to the needs. In this sense, the procedure they use is derived from the trimmed-toe transfer described by Wei and colleagues.[13] Other alternatives (eg, the second toe) provide a narrower and flimsier neothumb. The authors think that except in bilateral metacarpal hands, the second toe is a poor option even for children. In severe mutilating injuries that need more than one toe, the authors transplant the hallux as a first step. A week later, they carry out the reconstruction of the fingers with toes from the other foot. The authors have not had any untoward effect from such a short

delay, and this allows the patient to have the reconstruction done in one shot and start the rehabilitation without delay. Severe injuries need a plan for saving structures so that the surgeon might build an acceptable hand from scratch (**Fig. 9**). The authors have defined this ideal scenario — the acceptable hand — as one that has 3 fingers of the correct length with motion at the PIP joint, sensibility preserved, and a thumb.[5,14] When this is not possible, a tripod pinch is the minimum to be sought (**Fig. 10**).

The dissection of the toe is similar to that described in the Intercalated Defects section. It starts from the vein, which is traced to the proximal aspect of the flap. The artery is also located at the proximal edge of the toe and traced proximally. Usually the authors only include the digital artery, so they are not worried whether the first dorsal metatarsal is a plantar or dorsal type. By terminating the dissection at the take off point from the metatarsal vessels, the

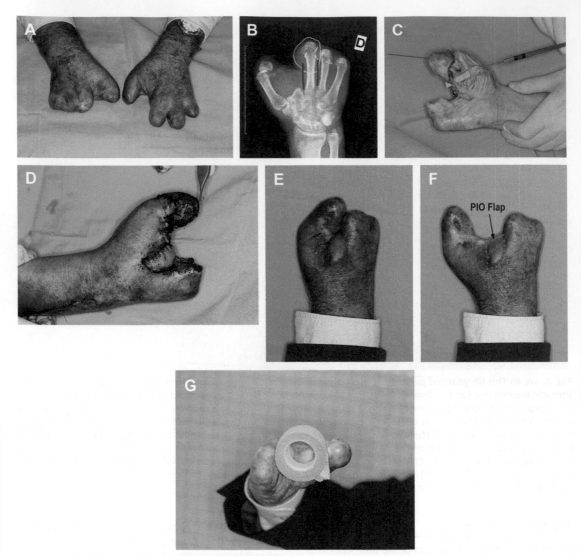

Fig. 8. (*A*) This 56-year-old patient was seen 1.5 years after sustaining bilateral below-the-knee amputations and loss of all digits after being critically ill due to a septic shock. Resection of both second metacarpals was done elsewhere several months later in an attempt to improve the first web space and the function. When first seen, he had no grasp or pinch with the too short right thumb except for using the thumb as a pusher for dialing on a specially designed cell phone display. (*B*) The plan was made to transfer the third metacarpal on both common digital arteries and nerves. (*C*) During surgery, the second common digital vessel was found to be scarred and hence useless. Only the third common digital vessel could be used to pedicle the stump. (*D*) To replace the scarred web and provide healthy tissue, a posterior interosseous flap was elevated concomitantly. (*E–G*) The ability to grab small- and medium-sized objects (including the handle of a crutch) was restored. (Copyright © 2016 Dr Piñal.)

surgeon will have enough length to perform a comfortable end-to-end anastomosis to the ulnar digital artery at the base of the thumb. If the base of the thumb is scarred, rather than going to the radial artery at the snuff-box, the authors prefer to dissect the radial digital artery of the index and flip it to the base of thumb. In this manner, the dissection of the foot is kept

to a minimum. This policy has the further advantage of allowing a much faster dissection in both hand and foot, but one has to be prepared to deal with vessels of a smaller diameter. Some tips have been given in Intermediate Defects section.

Toe-to-hand transfer in expert hands is an extremely reliable and safe procedure. In a

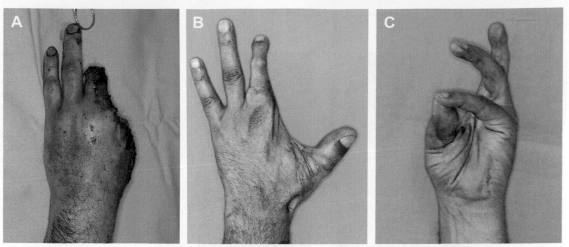

Fig. 9. (*A*) This patient lost the thumb and index at distal metacarpal level, and the middle finger at the proximal phalanx level. The hand was reconstructed by a trimmed toe and a second toe. Shape and acceptable function were reestablished as can be seen in these 15-year follow-up pictures (*B* and *C*). (Copyright © 2016 Dr Piñal.)

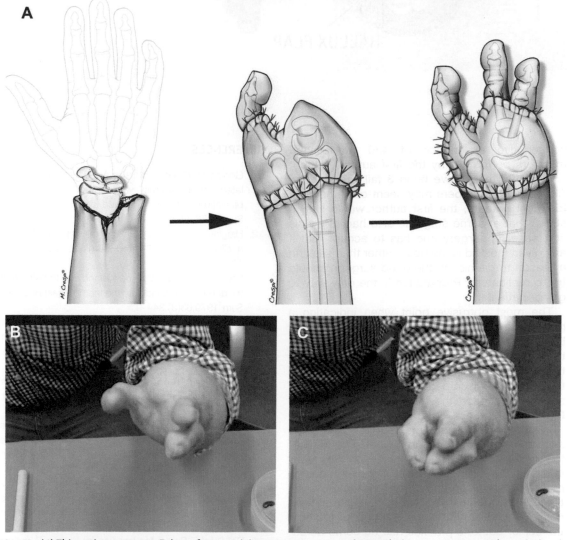

Fig. 10. (*A*) This patient was seen 5 days after sustaining a complex injury that ended in amputation at the wrist level. As an emergency the stump had been covered with a pedicled groin flap. In 2 stages, separated by 1 week, a tripod pinch was reconstructed. In the first stage, a second toe was planted in the radius (Furnas-Vilkki procedure),[15,16] and a free groin flap was used for cover. In the second stage, a combined second–third toe was transplanted on the lunate (*B* and *C*). The patient is able to grasp small objects to a 4 cm tripod pinch aperture. (Copyright © 2016 Dr Piñal.)

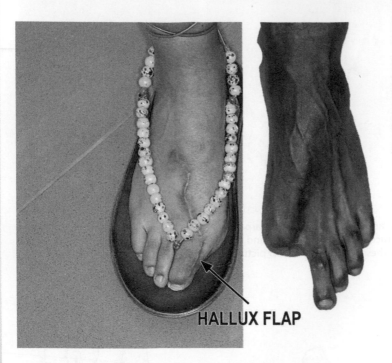

HALLUX FLAP

Fig. 11. Donor site after transposition of the proximal phalanx of the second toe on top of the base of the proximal phalanx of the hallux. Notice the flap to increase the girth of the transferred toe. On the right, the donor site of patient shown in **Fig. 9** that predated the introduction of the new technique of foot closure. (Copyright © 2016 Dr Piñal.)

consecutive experience of 420 toe-to-hand transfers performed by the first author, without exclusions, there have been 3 failures to date. Although the numbers may seem overwhelming for most readers, the first author would like to stress that at some stage he also had to do his first case. In surgery one has to accept that if any given method is the best, rather than seeking a reason to dismiss it, the good surgeon should try to replicate it. Preparation is the only way to go for patients.

The most obtrusive point when indicating a hallux is donor site morbidity, cosmetic deformity being so particularly obvious. To overcome this, the authors described a method where the second toe is transferred to the position of the hallux, and they used the discarded flap to reduce the hallux size and increase the girth of the second toe **Fig. 11**.[17]

In summary, despite the fact that there are several methods of thumb reconstruction, only toe transfer is ideal in the authors' view. Very rarely in the authors' practice does a patient decline reconstruction with a toe. For those rare cases, the authors offer them pollicization, or alternatively coverage with a Littler-type island flap. Never in the senior author's practice has he come across a case where the indication was a metacarpal lengthening.

REFERENCES

1. Godina M, Bajec J, Baraga A. Salvage of the mutilated upper extremity with temporary ectopic implantation of the undamaged part. Plast Reconstr Surg 1986;78(3):295–9.
2. Higgins JP. Ectopic banking of amputated parts: a clinical review. J Hand Surg Am 2011;36(11): 1868–76.
3. Foucher G, Braun JB. A new island flap transfer from the dorsum of the index to the thumb. Plast Reconstr Surg 1979;63(3):344–9.
4. Rose EH. Local arterialized island flap coverage of difficult hand defects preserving donor digit sensibility. Plast Reconstr Surg 1983;72(6): 848–58.
5. del Piñal F. The indications for toe transfer after "minor" finger injuries. J Hand Surg Br 2004;29(2): 120–9.
6. del Piñal F, García-Bernal FJ, Regalado J, et al. The tibial second toe vascularized neurocutaneous free flap for major digital nerve defects. J Hand Surg Am 2007;32(2):209–17.
7. del Piñal F, García-Bernal FJ, Delgado J, et al. Vascularized bone blocks from the toe phalanx to solve complex intercalated defects in the fingers. J Hand Surg Am 2006;31(7):1075–82.
8. Del Piñal F. Partial toe transfer. In: Slutsky D, editor. The art of microsurgical hand reconstruction. New York: Thiem; 2013. p. 420–6.

9. del Piñal F, García-Bernal FJ, Cagigal L, et al. Late salvage of the ischemic finger after crush injury using flow-through flaps: case report. J Hand Surg Am 2009;34(3):453–7.

10. Littler JW. The neurovascular pedicle method of digital transposition for reconstruction of the thumb. Plast Reconstr Surg 1953;12(5):303–19.

11. Ishida O, Taniguchi Y, Sunagawa T, et al. Pollicization of the index finger for traumatic thumb amputation. Plast Reconstr Surg 2006;117(3): 909–14.

12. Del Piñal F, Moraleda E, de Piero GH, et al. Onycho-osteo-cutaneous defects of the thumb reconstructed by partial hallux transfer. J Hand Surg Am 2014; 39(1):29–36.

13. Wei FC, Chen HC, Chuang CC, et al. Reconstruction of the thumb with a trimmed-toe transfer technique. Plast Reconstr Surg 1988;82: 506–15.

14. del Piñal F. Severe mutilating injuries to the hand: guidelines for organizing the chaos. J Plast Reconstr Aesthet Surg 2007;60(7):816–27.

15. Furnas DW, Achauer BM. Microsurgical transfer of the great toe to the radius to provide prehension after partial avulsion of the hand. J Hand Surg Am 1983;8(4):453–60.

16. Vilkki SK. Free toe transfer to the forearm stump following wrist amputation a current alternative to the Krukenberg operation. Handchir Mikrochir Plast Chir 1985;17:92e7 [in German].

17. del Piñal F, García-Bernal FJ, Regalado J, et al. A technique to improve foot appearance after trimmed toe or hallux harvesting. J Hand Surg Am 2007;32(3):409–13.

Secondary Thumb Reconstruction in a Mutilated Hand

David Graham, MBBS, FRACS(Orth), FAOrthA[a],
Praveen Bhardwaj, MS (Ortho), DNB (Ortho), FNB (Hand & Microsurgery), EDHS[b],
S. Raja Sabapathy, MS (Gen), MCh (Plastic), DNB (Plastic), FRCS (Edin), MAMS[c],*

KEYWORDS

- Thumb reconstruction • Osteoplastic reconstruction • Toe transfer • Pollicization

KEY POINTS

- The thumb plays a key role in global hand function.
- The reconstructed thumb requires length, sensation, stability, and the ability to meet the other digits, ideally in a tripod pinch.
- In secondary reconstruction of thumb in a mutilated hand, special consideration must be placed on the function of the remaining digits and allowing for functional pinch between the thumb and finger(s).
- Toe transfer remains the gold standard even in secondary reconstruction; osteoplastic thumb reconstruction and pollicization have a role and can provide useful function.

BACKGROUND

A mutilated hand is a devastating injury and a therapeutic challenge for the treating hand surgeon. A detailed history and examination needs to be performed, focusing on the patient's needs, hand dominance, occupation, hobbies, goals, and psychological state. A detailed assessment of what structures are missing and what are present is essential, including the bones, and soft tissues (muscles, tendons, blood vessels, and nerves). Setting realistic goals is imperative and having the patient participate in decision making may encourage acceptance of the injury. Ideally, the hand should be useful and aesthetically acceptable to the patient.

Most surgeons consider the goal in reconstruction in the multiple digit amputation to be a tripod grip rather than a basic grip, in which at least 2 fingers are in contact with the thumb, which gives rise to a stronger and more stable grip and pinch.

It is imperative that the hand surgeon considers not only the status of the thumb but also of the remaining digits. Littler[1] commented that "It is not the full length of the thumb, nor its great strength and movement, but rather its strategic position relative to the fingers and the integrity of the specialized terminal pulp tissue which determines prehensile status." Reflecting these comments, the specific reconstruction for an individual may need to be tailored to accommodate their specific injury.

In cases of significant hand trauma resulting in a mutilated hand, the surgeon must plan judiciously the appropriate treatment keeping in mind the overall goals. The reconstructed hand would preferably be pain free, have sensate tips, be stable, allow functional pinch and tripod grips, and be cosmetically acceptable.

[a] Department of Plastic, Hand & Reconstructive Microsurgery and Burns, Ganga Hospital, 313, Mettupalayam Road, Coimbatore 641 043, Tamil Nadu, India; [b] Hand & Wrist Surgery and Reconstructive Microsurgery, Ganga Hospital, 313, Mettupalayam Road, Coimbatore, Tamil Nadu 641 043, India; [c] Division of Plastic Surgery, Hand Surgery, Reconstructive Microsurgery and Burns, Ganga Hospital, 313, Mettupalayam Road, Coimbatore, Tamil Nadu 641 043, India
* Corresponding author.
E-mail address: rajahand@gmail.com

Hand Clin 32 (2016) 533–547
http://dx.doi.org/10.1016/j.hcl.2016.07.005
0749-0712/16/© 2016 Elsevier Inc. All rights reserved.

CLASSIFICATIONS

When assessing a patient with an amputated thumb multiple aspects must be considered. First, the remaining length of the thumb should be assessed. Lister[2] classified thumb defects into 4 groups based on the remaining length:

1. Acceptable length with poor soft tissue coverage,
2. Subtotal amputation with questionable remaining length,
3. Total amputation with preservation of the basal joint, and
4. Total amputation with loss of the basal joint.

This classification has implications for the options available for reconstruction. When assessing a patient with a mutilated hand, not only does the level of the thumb amputation need to be considered, but also of the status of the remaining digits, in consideration for restoring a tripod pinch grip. First, we deal with the status of the thumb.

There have been several other classification systems developed attempting to classify the mutilated hand. Wei and colleagues[3] proposed a classification of the metacarpal hand, and also discussed guidelines for management. This classification consists of 2 main categories, which are determined by the condition of the thumb. This is subdivided in to 1A, 1B, and 1C and 2A, 2B, and 2C, depending on the amputation level either middle proximal phalanx, metacarpophalangeal joint, or distal metacarpal respectively for the fingers or metacarpophalangeal joint, mid metacarpal, or proximal metacarpal, respectively, for the thumb.

Vilkki[4] proposed a classification for the no-finger hand in 2001. Level A refers to a 'basic hand' where there are a minimum of 2 functioning digital metacarpophalangeal joints and the thumb is amputated at the metacarpophalangeal joint or distal metacarpal level. This level has a good functional potential as there is no requirement for a metatarsophalangeal joint in reconstruction, thus making the reconstruction of a sound pinch or grip function easier. Level B is a true metacarpal hand with only a functional first metacarpal stump as a movable component. The Vilkki classification B includes both 2B and 2C of the Wei classification and can therefore be divided further into B1 with and B2 without adequate thenar musculature. The status of the adductor is of particular importance in evaluating the thenar muscles, because this is the most difficult function to reconstruct with tendon transfers. Level C is transcarpal and level D is more proximal—at the wrist or distal antebrachial amputation.

Tan and colleagues[5] reported on a case of bilateral metacarpal hand requiring reconstruction. The authors proposed reconstructing a tripod pinch for the dominant hand and a pulp to pulp pinch for the nondominant hand in type 2 metacarpal hand. A maximum of 5 toes were used in these transfers to avoid donor site complications.

Kotkansalo and colleagues[6] reviewed 8 patients (11 transfers) for posttraumatic metacarpal hand toe transfers at an average of 12 years of follow-up. All bar 1 patient were either satisfied or highly satisfied. Patients' perception of activities of daily living was generally good with many activities causing no difficulty or only slight difficulty. The authors concluded that it is possible to reconstruct a reasonable grip using microvascular toe transfers.

Group 1

Group 1 amputations rarely result in a functional deficit and may be termed a "compensated amputation." These patients require a sensate and supple tip, which can be provided by glabrous and nonglabrous skin flaps. These include the Moberg, V–Y advancement, neurovascular island (Littler) flap, free toe pulp transfer, first dorsal metacarpal artery (Foucher), cross finger, dorsoulnar/dorsoradial, and distant or free flaps, such as the posterior interosseous artery, reverse radial forearm, and free groin flaps (**Figs. 1–4**).

Group 2

It is generally accepted that amputation at the level of the proximal end of the proximal phalanx inevitability results in reduced hand span, difficulty in grasping large objects, and fine pinch limitations. Parvizi and colleagues[7] showed that proximal phalanx amputations that were not reconstructed resulted in poorer M2-DASH scores at midterm follow-up.

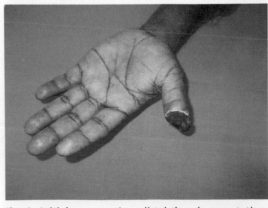

Fig. 1. Initial presentation: distal thumb amputation.

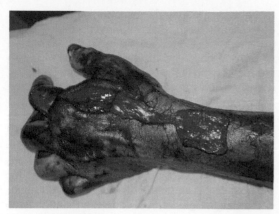

Fig. 2. Intraoperative photograph: Raising of the first dorsal metacarpal artery flap.

Distal proximal phalanx amputations often suffice with web deepening procedures. "Phalangization" are procedures that provide relative lengthening, without true lengthening and use either local, regional, distant pedicled, or free flaps.

Group 3

Untreated amputations at this level universally result in significant impairment. In the isolated thumb amputation setting, reconstructive options include osteoplastic reconstruction, distraction osteogenesis, pollicization, and free toe transfer variants.

Group 4

Absence of the basal joint proves difficult to treat, with limited available reconstructive options. The workhorse is in this group is pollicization, because this is the only option that will recreate a basal joint—the index metacarpophalangeal joint becoming the carpometacarpal joint of the new thumb. In the setting of a mutilated 'metacarpal' hand, pollicization is not possible. Hofer and

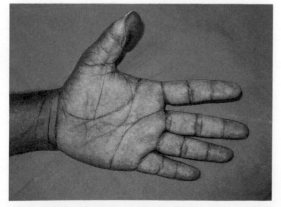

Fig. 3. The result at 6 months postoperative of a first dorsal metacarpal artery flap.

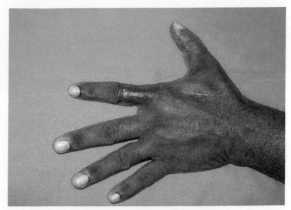

Fig. 4. The result at 6 months postoperative of a first dorsal metacarpal artery flap. The donor site grafted and healed well.

colleagues[8] recommended transplanting the ring finger of the uninjured hand to the annular finger position. Despite fantastic long-term results, this is not a routinely accepted practice. Although this has not been described in the literature, it this may be an option for a metacarpal hand with absence of the thumb basal joint.

TOE TRANSFER

Toe transfer is a fantastic option for amputations distal to the carpometacarpal joint, providing the most reliable cosmetic and functional outcome. The procedure, however, requires microsurgical expertise. When a future toe transfer is being considered, a local or regional flap is not advisable during the index procedure, because this may damage the critical vascular network. A pedicled groin flap is an excellent option in this situation. Harvesting the toe with the metatarsal requires soft tissue coverage, almost always necessitating a preliminarily groin flap. Sabapathy and colleagues[9] reviewed 8 cases of second toe transfer, all of which underwent a preliminary groin flap. In this series, all patients achieved opposition. The authors commented that the flap should point in the direction of the new thumb, and should be of sufficient length, because short flaps limit the length of metatarsal that can be taken. They found that attention to detail with flap coverage, optimizing function of the remaining digits and strategic positioning of the transferred toe were essential for a good outcome.

Great Toe

The great toe flap is based on either the dorsal or plantar metatarsal artery and is harvested along with the dorsal venous network, and deep peroneal and digital nerves. Several modifications have been advocated, motivated by donor site morbidity and the 20% discrepancy in size of the thumb and great toe.[10] When multiple digits are injured, the great toe is preferred to a second toe, because the second toe may not adequately recreate powerful pinch grip.

TRIMMED TOE

A trimmed toe transfer was described by Wei and colleagues[11] in which a longitudinal osteotomy is performed to thin the toe to replicate the native thumb size and also maintaining some interphalangeal joint movement.

WRAP AROUND TOE

Morrison and colleagues[12] described the wrap-around flap, which uses the great toe pulp, nail and a segment of distal phalanx, which is transferred with an iliac crest bone graft. This procedure results in improved cosmesis of the donor and recipient sites; however, this improvement is at the expense of no interphalangeal joint movement. The graft is also subject to resorption.

SECOND TOE

Because the second toe is not critical during the gait cycle, it allows for the entire metatarsophalangeal joint to be harvested. Therefore, this may be the only toe transfer possible for proximal thumb amputations. Criticisms include a poorer cosmetic appearance, a tendency to claw, and a short nail.

Owing to anatomic or cultural reasons, free toe transfer is occasionally not a possibility. Alternatively, osteoplastic reconstruction, pollicization, or lengthening may be considered. Metacarpal lengthening via distraction osteogenesis was described by Matev[13]; however, it only yields approximately 3 cm of length and although this is still beneficial, better alternatives usually exist. Other limitations include prolonged length of the treatment, poor cosmesis, and lack of movement.

The mainstay of treatment of a mutilated 'metacarpal hand' has been multiple toe transfers. How many toes, which toes, when to perform and where to place them is controversial. Multiple toe transfer for reconstruction of a mutilated hand is not a recent advance. Borovikov[14] described a split great toe in block with the second toe reconstructing a thumb and index finger reconstruction. In the same year, Yu-dong and colleagues[15] also used a monoblock transfer of a wrap around flap from the great toe (and an iliac crest graft) along with the second toe. In 2002, Chang and Jones[16] harvested the great and second toes in block.

Wei and colleagues[17] described a case report of a mutilated hand that underwent multiple toe transfers. Initially, a pedicled groin flap was used to provide coverage of the thumb stump and to reconstruct the first web, then a combined second and third toe transfer was used to recreate the amputated index and middle fingers. A second toe was used to reconstruct the thumb, and an iliac osteocutaneous flap for reconstruction of the ulna border of the palm.

The same group in 1998[18] examined the success rates of combined second and third toes for multiple digital amputation in the mutilated hand, comparing single versus double arterial anastomosis of 57 transfers. In the single anastomosis group, 10 of 41 (24.4%) required re-exploration with an overall 92.7% success rate, compared with 1 of 16 (6.2%) in the double anastomosis group; the overall success rate was 100%.

In a similar setting, Del Piñal and colleagues[19] reported on the use of combined second and third toe transfer for reconstruction of a traumatic metacarpal hand. The authors noted an overall survival rate of 94 of 95 toe transfers. Of these, 5 patients had sustained amputations of all 5 digits (3 cases) and 4 digits (2 cases). These patients underwent combined second and third toe flap transplants. The thumb was reconstructed by a great toe transfer in 4 of the thumb amputations and by an emergency ectopic middle finger reimplantation in 1 case. They considered thumb reconstruction a priority and performed this 1 week before the dual transplant. They used dual arterial anastomosis in 3 cases and three arterial anastomoses in 1. The authors reported a 100% survival rate; however, re-exploration was required in 2 cases. All patients were noted to obtain a stable tripod pincer grip. All patients were satisfied with the result, and there were no complications of toe crossover or painful gait reported. The authors classified the injuries into 3 groups. Type I involved all triphalangeal fingers are missing, type II the radial digits are missing, and type III all digits, including the thumb are missing.

In another case series, Chung and Kotsis[20] reported on 2 farmers who sustained amputations of all digits and underwent a 3-toe transfer from both feet. The first patient underwent preliminary groin flap for soft tissue coverage, a delayed second toe to thumb transfer, and a subsequent combined contralateral second and third toe transfer to the middle and ring finger positions to achieve tripod pinch. At 4 years of follow-up, the total active ranges of motion for the thumb, index, and middle fingers were 71°, 72°, and 82°, respectively, with excellent sensory return noted by Semmes Weinstein monofilament testing. He was able to return to full duties, including no pain on walking. The second patient underwent local flaps for primary coverage owing to the digits not being salvageable. At 5 months after injury, he underwent ipsilateral second toe transfer to reconstruct the thumb. Five months later, he underwent contralateral second and third toe transfer to reconstruct the middle and ring fingers. At 2 years of follow-up, he was able to operate machinery and had a Semmes Weinstein score of 3.61 for all transferred toes. Total active motion was 65°, 66°, and 60° for the middle finger, ring finger, and thumb, respectively (normal, 260°).

Julve and Villen[21] reported on 10 cases of either traumatic loss or congenital deficiency who underwent monoblock transfer of the great and second toes. The authors performed a total of 56 toe to hand transfers, of which 10 were performed as a monoblock, and 8 of these incorporating the great and second toes. The majority (9 of 10) were for traumatic amputation. Interestingly, they reported superior results in the traumatic patients compared with the congenital deficiency case. Donor site problems were reported to be tolerable and transient. Eight of the 10 cases developed a 2-point discrimination satisfactory for protective sensation. The authors always maintained the proximal phalanx of the great toe and the second toe when possible to maintain a proper toe-off gait. They noted on average a 2.5-hour increase in operating time over a single toe transfer, but a 40% reduction in time over 2 separate toe transfers. The authors commented that to minimize the risk of losing 2 toes, they ensured there are 2 arterial anastomoses, and also included more venous anastomoses than for a single transfer.

Venkatramani and colleagues[22] recently reported on 11 patients who underwent free toe transfer to reconstruct posttraumatic metacarpal hands. They concluded that even a single toe transfer may restore useful function. The authors commented that the ultimate success of a metacarpal hand reconstruction is determined by the very first operation the patient undergoes. Ideally, every effort should be made to preserve bone length, in particular, to spare the metacarpophalangeal joints of the fingers or interphalangeal joint of the thumb. The residual joint will improve the mobility of a future toe transfer and allow greater functional dexterity. The authors concluded that even a single toe transfer can result in satisfactory results in these situations, with all patients achieving 'good' results and being satisfied with their outcome. The authors also noted that sensory recovery in the transferred toes steadily improves with time, sometimes taking several years. This is often reflected in Semmes Weinstein monofilament tests, although not in terms of static or moving 2-point discrimination.

MULTIPLE TOE TRANSFERS
How Many Toes to Transfer? Two or Three?

Obviously, there is less donor morbidity and is technically less demanding when harvesting fewer toes. Transferring 3 rather than 2 toes allow recreation of tripod pinch, and a resulting a larger surface contact area for pulp to pulp pinch increasing grip strength. Wei advocated the use of multiple toe transfers to recreate a tripod pinch, Venkatramani and colleagues[22] reported in their series that even though reconstruction with multiple toes may have functional and aesthetic advantages, the donor defect on the foot is considerably greater. In their population who frequently wear sandals, this is often too difficult for a patient to accept.

Where to Put the Toes?

When deciding where to place the transplanted toes it is important to remember that the toes must be able to comfortably reach the thumb to allow pinch tripod grip. When the toes are placed in the position of the ring and small fingers, this may result in digits too short to reach the thumb. In contrast, when placed in the position of the index and middle finger positions, this may result in a hand with a reduced span and hence difficulty in holding larger objects. Therefore, the usual choice is to transfer the toes to the middle and ring ringer positions to avoid these problems.

In contrast with this approach, Wallace and Wei[23] commented that, after the thumb, the radial 2 digits play the dominant role in global hand function (in most patients), with the exception of a few who require a larger hand span. They therefore felt that these should be reconstructed preferentially. The authors also commented that when reconstructing amputations distal to the web space, it is preferable to perform 2 separate toe harvests to preserve a deep webspace; however, the more proximal amputations may be reconstructed with a monoblock transfer of the second/third or third/fourth toes on a single vascular pedicle.

Venkatramani and colleagues,[22] who advocated a single toe transfer suggested that when a single toe is transferred, it is more cosmetically appealing when placed on the radial or ulna border of the hand compared with being placed centrally. The authors' preferred position for a single toe transfer (in most patients) is at the index finger position. When 2 toes are to be transferred, they prefer to transfer the great toe first, and once this is moving freely, they then decide on the optimal position for the second toe to allow a full pinch.

Specific Considerations in Secondary Thumb Reconstruction in the Mutilated Hand

Some physicians have advocated a below elbow amputation and fitting of a prosthesis in these cases; however, 38% of patients in a study[24] abandoned use of their prosthesis owing to limited usefulness, and hence at this stage biological reconstructive options, although not perfect, usually provide a more satisfactory outcome. Hand transplantation has also gained interest around the world for these injuries; however, given the potential for rejection and requirement of immunosuppression, this has not become widely accepted, except in unique situations, such as in meningococcal septicemia resulting in bilateral hand loss and renal failure requiring transplantation.

In an effort to recreate this, the combined second and third toe free transfer was described. This transfer is the workhorse transfer for multiple digit amputations proximal to the commissural fold.

Multiple classification systems have been proposed for the traumatic metacarpal hand. The definition is also debated. Michon and Dolich[25] defined it as a hand that has no prehensile ability except to function as a hook. In contrast, Wei and associates[3] defined a metacarpal hand as one where all fingers have been amputated proximal to the middle third of the proximal phalanx. He subclassified it into 2 groups: type I, where the thumb is present; and type II, where the thumb has been amputated. Del Piñal and associates[19] proposed another classification in an attempt to minimize confusion: in type I, the thumb is present; in type II, only 1 triphalangic digit remains; and in type III, all digits have been amputated.

Again, there remains controversy surrounding the specific preferred technique to reconstruct the posttraumatic metacarpal hand. Wei and Del Piñal advocated the combined second/third toe transfer; however, Foucher[26] considers that the double toe flap should never be performed owing to the donor site morbidity; instead, elective toe transfer of 1 toe from each foot is preferred. When the thumb also requires reconstruction (a true metacarpal hand), Foucher prefers to achieve a basic grip (with 1 toe from each foot) or uses a prosthesis.

SURGICAL OPTIONS: THE THUMB

Although microsurgical free toe transfer is the most common method for thumb reconstruction, there are several other alternatives that may be of more use in specific injuries.

On Top Plasty/Ectopic Replantation

Whenever confronted with a mutilated hand, an important principle not to be forgotten is that of 'spare parts surgery.' Occasionally, a digit may not be replantable in its native position; however, it may be used in a purposefully chosen ectopic position, whereby a partial thumb amputation gains length by the addition of an amputated digit.

Osteoplastic Reconstruction

Reconstruction of the thumb by microsurgical techniques by toe transfers remains the gold standard. Occasionally, situations arise and this is not possible, or microsurgical expertise is not available. In this situation, conventional osteoplastic thumb reconstruction is the best choice. Osteoplastic reconstruction has the advantage of not sacrificing other digits, is a relatively quick procedure and the sensation is immediate (with an added Littler flap) in contrast with a toe transfer. Attention to detail is paramount when aiming for a good outcome, just as when performing a microsurgical toe transfer. Sabapathy and colleagues[27] had a rare opportunity to perform a great toe transfer on the nondominant thumb and osteoplastic thumb reconstruction on the dominant thumb in a case of a student who sustained a bilateral thumb amputation. This unique case resulted in an opportunity to directly compare the techniques in the same individual. At the 15-year follow-up, he was extremely happy with the functional status of the osteoplastic thumb for the dominant right side. He reported no difficulty, even when performing fine pinch activities (**Figs. 5–12**).

Osteoplastic thumb reconstruction essentially involves creating a skin tube out of a pedicled groin flap and at a later stage introduction of a

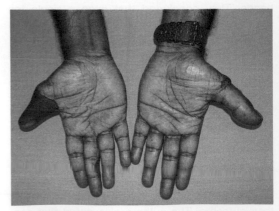

Fig. 5. At the 15-year follow-up of bilateral thumb amputations. The right hand was reconstructed with an osteoplastic technique and left with a great toe to thumb transfer.

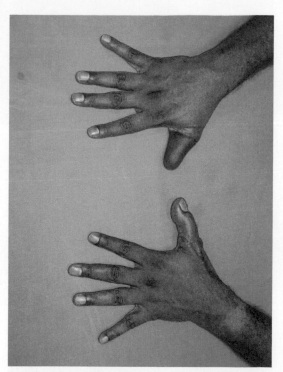

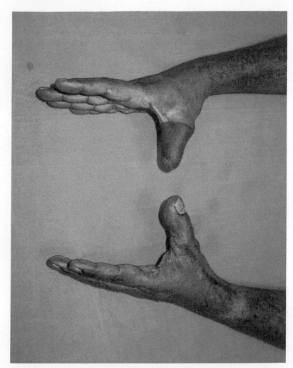

Fig. 6. At the 15-year follow-up. Functional comparison of osteoplastic reconstruction (*right hand*) and great toe transfer (*left hand*).

Fig. 8. At the 15-year follow-up. Functional comparison of osteoplastic reconstruction (*right hand*) and great toe transfer (*left hand*).

nonvascularized bone graft for stability and Littler's island flap for sensation. Following certain technical points help to result in a satisfactory outcome.

Most often, a groin flap is the flap of choice, which is tubed during attachment. The line of attachment is oblique to increase the extent of skin inset, and it is attached in such a way that the tube points out in the direction of the normal thumb. If the tube points in another direction, it is difficult at a later stage to correct, and even though

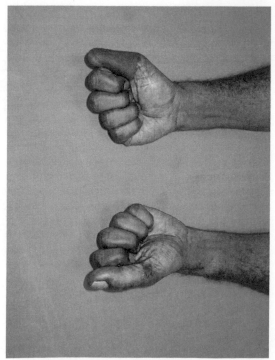

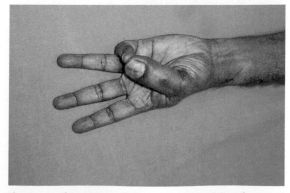

Fig. 7. At the 15-year follow-up. Functional comparison of osteoplastic reconstruction (*right hand*) and great toe transfer (*left hand*).

Fig. 9. At the 15-year follow-up. Opposition function of the great toe transfer.

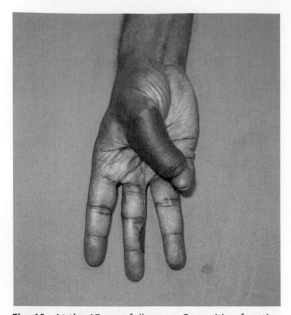

Fig. 10. At the 15-year follow-up. Opposition function of the osteoplastic reconstruction.

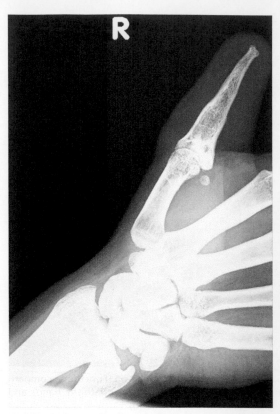

Fig. 12. Radiograph of osteoplastic thumb reconstruction at 15 years postoperative.

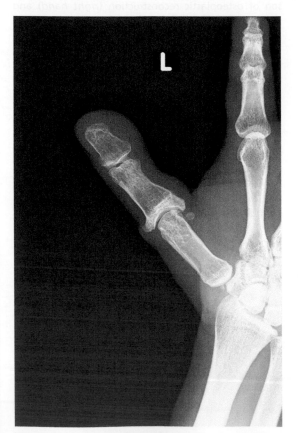

Fig. 11. Radiograph of great toe to thumb reconstruction at 15 years postoperative.

it may be possible to complete the reconstruction, the cosmetic result is suboptimal. The distal portion of the groin flap has a random blood supply and this is the portion that will be most relevant during reconstruction. This portion of the graft may be significantly thinned to achieve a better cosmetic result. Divergent views exist as to the side of the suture line; it may be placed either on the outer or inner side. The authors prefer to keep the suture line on the inner side, because it can be opened if required be when performing the next stage, namely, a Littler's island neurovascular flap and bone grafting. We have also attempted to introduce the bone graft during the time of flap; however, this practice does not seem to yield any advantage. Even if the bone is introduced in the primary setting, the patient will still require another procedure to provide sensation in the form of Littler's neurovascular island flap. Therefore, we find it better, to combine the bone graft and neurovascular island flap.

Once attached the flap is subjected to a delay procedure before division. Many groin flaps to the hand can safely be divided without a delay. This would depend on the extent of skin attachment. In a tubed flap, the length of attachment in relation to the flap size is relatively small and hence it is mandatory to perform a delay procedure before flap division. If not performed, there is a risk of partial flap loss, which one can ill afford when performing a secondary reconstruction. We delay the flap at 3 weeks, by partial division of the flap at the base and divide the axial vessel if one is able to visualize it. The skin is then resutured. The flap is completely divided 1 week after the delay procedure.

The next stage of bone grafting and island flap can be done anytime after 6 weeks after division of the flap. We prefer an iliac crest bone graft, and a good portion of corticocancellous graft is harvested. It is important to have some element of cortical graft to reduce the extent of resorption. Usually, the osteoplastic thumb reconstruction is undertaken for thumb loss at the metacarpophalangeal or distal metacarpal level. The harvested bone graft is pegged into the metacarpal and secure fixation is obtained by a screw or more often by an axial Kirchner wire. Originally the island flap procedure was performed a few months after the bone grafting in another stage; however, we find it is preferable to undertake them together. This not only reduces cost and saves time in rehabilitation, but it also reduces the extent of bone resorption in the long term. In our experience, we have found that, if island flap is also undertaken concomitantly, bone resorption is lessened. This is likely owing to the presence of sensory feedback; as the amount of pressure loaded on the bone graft is more when there is no sensory feedback. It is well-known that, in the absence of sensation, the pressure on pinch is much greater than when the fingers are sensate.

The island flap is raised from the ulnar side of the middle finger. The size of the flap could be large or small; however, we now harvest a flap of approximately 3 cm in length. An elliptical flap of that length and extending from the midline on the volar side to the first third on the dorsal side is taken. It is essential that there is no tension on the neurovascular bundle after the inset of the flap into the thumb, even in the position of maximum stretch of the thumb, the vascular pedicle and the nerve must be lying comfortably. In some series, the long-term results of the 2PD obtained by the Littler island flap has decreased with time. This was an unexpected finding, which could be explained by the stretch of the nerve when the thumb moves into the limits of extension and abduction. The only way to reduce the tension is by obtaining a long length of the pedicle by proper planning of the flap. The distal flap edge is kept just proximal to the level of the germinal matrix of the nail. In this way, the flap will comfortably reach the destination. The donor site is covered with a full-thickness skin graft. An ellipse of flap skin is excised exactly at the contact surface of the neo thumb to the fingers. When the bone graft is harvested from the iliac crest, leaving a little soft tissue attached to the cortical side is useful so that, when the island flap is attached, a nonabsorbable suture can be used to fix the undersurface of the flap to the bone graft.

Osteoplastic reconstruction can also be performed using the reverse radial artery forearm flap. A segment of vascularized bone from the radius can be harvested with the flap. However, because the available bone is thin, bone from the iliac crest is taken as the graft and the flap wrapped around the bone graft. Littler's island flap can also be done at the same stage. One advantage of the radial artery forearm flap is the reduction in the number of stages. In the longer term however, patients are happier with the groin flap donor site, because it does not leave a scar in the forearm. Recently, a medial femoral condyle free flap has also been described in the setting of osteoplastic reconstruction.[28] Other drawbacks include poor cosmesis, cortical sensory integration, bone resorption, and the requirement for 2 procedures.

Functionally, the osteoplastic thumb performs well, but aesthetically it falls far short of a well-done toe transfer. It will continue to be used in difficult situations and it is essential that the surgeon is aware of the technical considerations that are important to achieve a good functional outcome (**Figs. 13–18**).

Pollicization

Pollicization is another reconstructive option. Often a thumb amputation also results in injury to the adjacent digits. Pollicization of an injured index finger not only provides length to the thumb, but

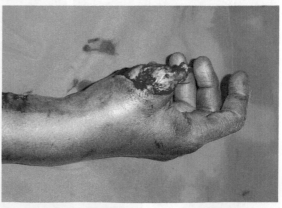

Fig. 13. Initial presentation of thumb amputation.

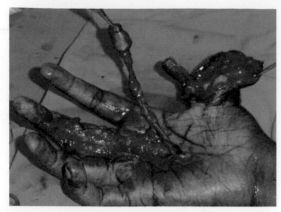

Fig. 14. Intraoperative photograph. Raising the Littler's neurovascular flap from the middle finger for thumb sensation.

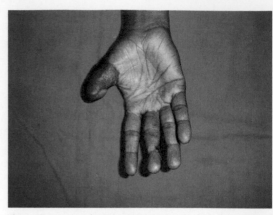

Fig. 17. Osteoplastic reconstruction. Final clinical result.

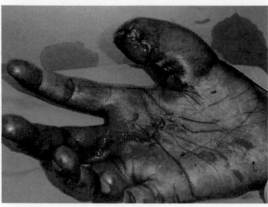

Fig. 15. Intraoperative photograph. Conclusion of the osteoplastic reconstruction with Littler's flap.

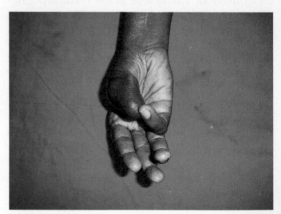

Fig. 18. Osteoplastic reconstruction. Final clinical result. The patient is able to oppose to the little finger.

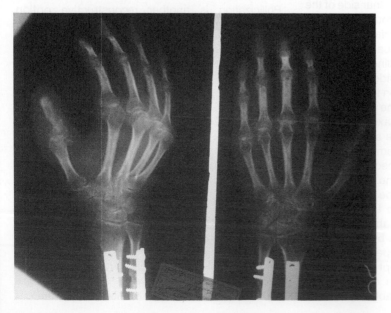

Fig. 16. Osteoplastic reconstruction radiographs.

also widens the webspace. Pollicization of the middle finger has been described in cases of injury to the thumb and index finger; however, using the index finger remains the standard and safer option.

Pollicization may not be practical owing to global hand injury; however, second toe transfer may still be possible. Lin and colleagues[29] preferred osteoplastic reconstruction when pollicization was not possible; however, of the 3 cases with loss of the carpometacarpal joint in their series, only 1 regained opposition.

Pollicization in the Setting of Secondary Reconstruction of Thumb

Politicization is the preferred method of thumb reconstruction for loss at the carpometacarpal joint level. Naturally, the availability of a finger that could be pollicized is a prerequisite for this procedure. Pollicization in the posttraumatic setting differs in several technical aspects from when it is performed in the congenital setting. First, the injury that results in total loss of the thumb also may have caused significant injury to the adjacent fingers and/or the palm. Loss of thenar muscles and segmental loss of long flexor and extensor tendons require tendon grafts or transfers in addition to pollicization. Another factor that we have noted is the need for flap cover to fill up the newly created thumb web. Usually, the radial border skin is too scarred to provide good flap coverage for the web space. After the pollicization, bare bone and critical structures would be exposed, and to maintain the integrity of the first web, a flap is required. The posterior interosseous artery flap admirably fills the requirement (**Figs. 19–24**).

Most commonly, the radial digital artery of the index finger would be injured concomitantly. Therefore, the finger needs to be mobilized solely on the ulnar side digital artery and utmost care needs to be exercised during its dissection. Because the ulnar artery is most often the

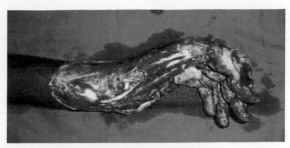

Fig. 20. After debridement, raw area was covered with a groin flap.

dominant arterial supply to the digit, this is usually sufficient. If the dorsum is scarred and veins are damaged, an alternate source of venous drainage needs to be planned during the mobilization of the finger. A strip of volar skin can be taken along with sufficient tissues for providing venous drainage and the finger pollicized (**Figs. 25–28**).

Most injuries that result in total loss of the thumb are associated with skin loss in the radial border of the hand. In the acute stage, skin grafts are not usually adequate to cover these defects. In planning for the future requirements, flap cover needs to be provided. We prefer either a free flap or a distant pedicled groin flap if the soft tissue defect is large. We wish to preserve the options of a posterior interosseous artery flap or reverse radial artery forearm flap for the reconstruction of the first web space and for the use of the vessels for any possible future microsurgical procedure.

Metacarpal Lengthening

Metacarpal lengthening has the advantage of retaining the native innervation; however, it requires a lengthy treatment duration and is undertaken infrequently. This is usually not the technique of choice for most reconstructions whether isolated thumb or for a thumb with a mutilated hand.

Timing of Reconstruction

Whether to undertake the definitive procedure as an acute or subacute procedure (ie, during the same hospitalization) remains controversial. Henry and Wei[30] noted that this may shorten convalescence and may be technically easier owing to avoiding the secondary scaring and fibrosis. Yim and colleagues[31] and Woo and colleagues[32] have each demonstrated no increased complications with early toe transfer over a delayed procedure.

For multiple reasons, a primary definitive procedure may not be feasible. When the amputated thumb is present, replantation must always be

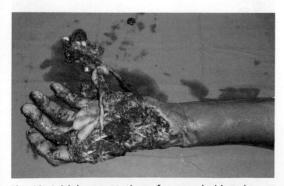

Fig. 19. Initial presentation of a mangled hand.

Graham et al

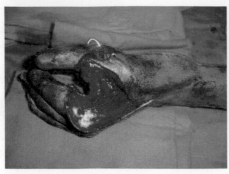
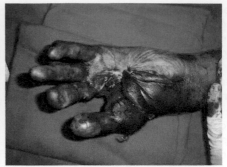

Fig. 21. At 3 months, the hand is reconstructed with a pollicization of the index finger. This left a defect in the first webspace.

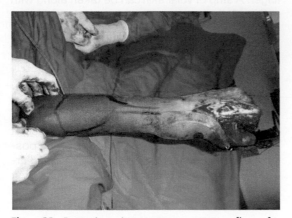

Fig. 22. Posterior interosseous artery flap for coverage of first web raw area.

attempted because no reconstructive procedure is superior to a successful replantation. Occasionally, this attempted replantation may prove to be unsuccessful despite promising early viability. The patient may not be medically stable for a prolonged procedure in the setting of multiple trauma, or may not be ready psychologically to accept the proposed treatments in the primary setting.

Increasing Length and Mobility

Although in the setting of isolated thumb amputation, distal third amputations may be

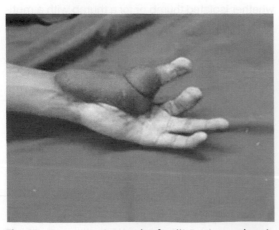

Fig. 23. Postoperative result of pollicization and groin flap.

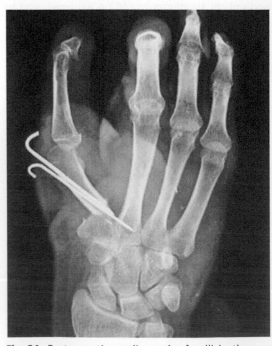

Fig. 24. Postoperative radiograph of pollicization.

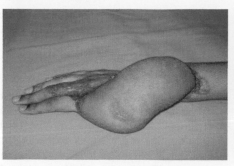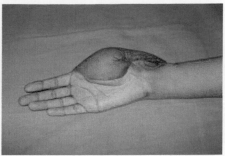

Fig. 25. Engineering student referred after anterolateral thigh flap and failed toe transfer. Note dorsal grafted area; no dorsal veins available.

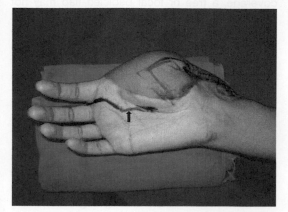

Fig. 26. Preoperative markings for pollicization.

well-accepted and often termed 'compensated amputations,' when multiple digits are injured this may not still be applicable.

Secondary Tendon Transfers

Despite optimal reconstructive procedures, it may still be necessary to undertake secondary tendon transfers. Proximal thumb amputations may have lost the intrinsic musculature needed for thumb adduction and opposition. In this situation, the options for reconstruction of opposition include extensor carpi radialis longus, palmaris longus, and ring finger flexor digitorum superficialis as donor tendon; the ultimate choice depends on what structures were also injured during the initial trauma. As mentioned, adductor function is the most difficult to reconstruct with tendon transfers.

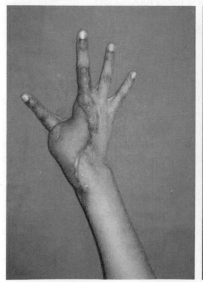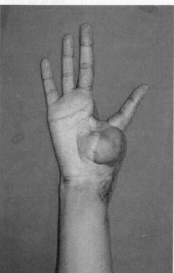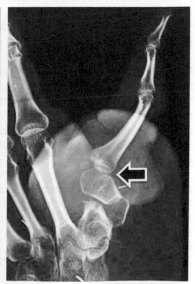

Fig. 27. Postpollicization clinical photos and radiograph. The CMC joint has been recreated from the MCP joint of the index finger (*arrow*). Note the extended position of the MCP joint to prevent hyper-extension of the recreated CMC joint.

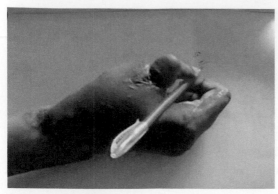

Fig. 28. Postpollicization. The patient is able to function well, including writing.

First Web Space Creation

When managing the mutilated hand with a deficient thumb, there are several instances when the first web space may be deficient. For a thumb amputation at the level of the proximal phalanx, often a 'phalangization' procedure designed to increase relative length of the thumb will suffice. At least one-half of the proximal phalanx is required to undertake phalangization along with minimal scarring and no web contracture. Flap options include Z-plasty (single, 4 or 5 flap), dorsal rotation, regional or free flaps (including posterior interosseous artery, reverse radial forearm, groin flap). Z-plasties are appropriate for deepening the web; however, regional or free flaps may be more beneficial when aiming for web widening. A 5 flap Z-plasty combines Z-plasties with a V–Y advancement flap.

A dorsal rotation flap may be used in cases of scarring or adduction contracture of the first web.

Second, when multiple digits are amputated in the setting of a mutilated hand, the first webspace may be inadequate to allow functional pinch. In this setting, 'on-top plasty' harvesting of the distal portion of the amputated index finger and placing it onto the amputated thumb stump addresses not only the lack of length of the thumb, but also increases the first web space.

Third, scar contracture may result in a poorly positioned thumb and limits the patients' function. When significant, a first web space release may greatly improve the overall hand function of the patient. The options for coverage in this setting include local, regional, distant, and free flaps. Skin grafts have a tendency to contract and therefore are best avoided. Locally, a dorsal rotation flap may be sufficient for mild to moderate contractures. For more severe contractures, a posterior interosseous artery flap, radial or ulna artery

forearm flaps, free lateral arm fasciocutaneous, or free groin flaps are often considered.

CONSIDERATIONS AT THE INDEX PROCEDURE

A mutilated hand may be an overwhelming presentation for the less experienced hand surgeon. It is essential to undertake an adequate radical debridement at the index procedure and provide soft tissue coverage to allow the underlying tendons and bones to glide in a minimally scarred bed. Leaving a poorly debrided wound or failing to provide adequate soft tissue coverage will ultimately result in a poor long-term result.

When there is significant tissue loss requiring coverage, a free or local pedicled flap may not be possible owing to potential damage to the local vessels. In this scenario, a pedicled flap based on the superficial circumflex iliac artery or superficial inferior epigastric artery is an excellent option for importing a soft and supple skin coverage, which may later require a secondary reconstructive procedure, such as a free toe transfer.

SUMMARY

Thumb reconstruction in the setting of a mutilated hand provides a particular challenge for the hand surgeon. Particular attention needs to be paid to the assessment of the remaining length and stability of the remaining thumb but also of the function of the remaining digits. The ultimate functional result depends greatly on the ability of the thumb to contact the remaining digit(s) and allow the patient to use the hand functionally.

REFERENCES

1. Littler JW. Finger pollicization for traumatic loss. In: McCarthy J, editor. Plastic Surgery: The Hand. Vol 8, Pt 2. Philadelphia: Saunders; 1990. p. 5135–52.
2. Lister G. The choice of procedure following thumb amputation. Clin Orthop Relat Res 1984;195:45–51.
3. Wei FC, El-Gammal TA, Lin CH, et al. Metacarpal hand: classification and guidelines for microsurgical reconstruction with toe transplants. Plast Reconstr Surg 1997;99:122–8.
4. Vilkki SK. Functional restoration of the no-finger hand. In: Duparc J, Alnot JY, Soucacos P, editors. Surgical techniques in orthopaedics and traumatology. Paris: Scientifiques et Mé;dicales Elsevier SAS; 2001. 55–390-B-10, 8p.
5. Jan DK, Wul FO, Lutz RS, et al. Strategies in multiple toe transplantation for bilateral type II metacarpal hand reconstruction. Hand Clin 1999;15:607–12.
6. Kotkansalo T, Vilkki SK, Elo P. The functional results of post-traumatic metacarpal hand reconstruction

with microvascular toe transfers. J Hand Surg Eur Vol 2009;34(6):730–42.

7. Parvizi D, Koch H, Friedl H, et al. Analysis of functional outcome after posttraumatic thumb reconstruction in comparison to non reconstructed amputated thumbs at the proximal phalanx of the thumb ray: a mid-term follow-up with special attention to the Manchester-modified M2 DASH questionnaire and effect size of Cohen's d. J Trauma 2012; 72(2):33–40.

8. Hofer SO, Cronin KJ, Morrison WA. A long-term study of ring finger transfer in the reconstruction of transmetacarpal amputations. J Hand Surg Am 2002;27A:1087–94.

9. Sabapathy SR, Venkatramani H, Bhardwaj P. Reconstruction of the thumb amputation at the carpometacarpal joint level by groin flap and second toe transfer. Injury 2013;44:370–5.

10. Pet MA, Ko JH, Vedder NB. Reconstruction of the traumatized thumb. Plast Reconstr Surg 2014; 134(6):1235–45.

11. Wei FC, Chen HC, Chuang CC, et al. Reconstruction of the thumb with a trimmed-toe transfer technique. Plast Reconstr Surg 1988;82:506–15.

12. Morrison WA, O'Brien BM, MacLeod AM. Thumb reconstruction with a free neurovascular wrap-around flap from the big toe. J Hand Surg Am 1980;5:575–83.

13. Matev IB. Thumb reconstruction through metacarpal bone lengthening. J Hand Surg Am 1980;5(5):482–7.

14. Borovikov A. Toe-to-hand transfers in the rehabilitation of frostbite injury. Ann Plast Surg 1993;31:245–50.

15. Yu-dong G, Gao-meng Z, De-shong C, et al. Free toe transfer for thumb and finger reconstruction in 300 cases. Plast Reconstr Surg 1993;91:693–702.

16. Chang J, Jones NF. Simultaneous toe-to-hand transfer and lower extremity amputations for severe upper and lower limb defects: the use of spare parts. J Hand Surg 2002;27B:219–23.

17. Wei FC, Seah CS, Chen HC, et al. Functional and esthetic reconstruction of a mutilated hand using multiple toe transfers and iliac osteocutaneous flap: a case report. Microsurgery 1993;14(6):388–90.

18. Cheng MH, Wei FC, Santamria E, et al. Single versus double arterial anastomoses in combined second – and third toe transplantation. Plast Reconstr Surg 1998;102(7):2408–12.

19. Del Piñal F, García-Bernal FJ, Delgado J, et al. Reconstruction of metacarpal hand by combined second and third toe transfer. Rev Esp Cir Ortop Traumatol 2007;51(1):15–24.

20. Chung KC, Kotsis SV. Outcomes of multiple microvascular toe transfers for reconstruction in 2 patients with digitless hands: 2- and 4-year follow-up case reports. J Hand Surg Am 2002;27A(4):652–8.

21. Julve GG, Villen GM. The multiple monoblock toe-to-hand transfer in digital reconstruction: a report of ten cases. J Hand Surg Br 2004;29B(3):220–7.

22. Venkatramani H, Bhardwaj P, Sierakowski A, et al. Functional outcomes of post-traumatic metacarpal hand reconstruction with free toe-to-hand transfer. Indian J Plast Surg 2016;49(1):16–25.

23. Wallace CG, Wei FC. Posttraumatic finger reconstruction with microsurgical transplantation of toes. Hand Clin 2007;23:117–28.

24. Wright TW, Hagen AD, Wood MB. Prosthetic usage in major upper extremity amputations. J Hand Surg 1995;20A:619–22.

25. Michon J, Dolich BH. The metacarpal hand. Hand 1974;6:285–90.

26. Foucher G. Discussion. Plast Reconstr Surg 1998; 102:2413.

27. Sabapathy SR, Venkatramani H, Bharathi RR. Functional evaluation of a great toe transfer and the osteoplastic technique for thumb reconstruction in the same individual. J Hand Surg Br 2003;28B(5): 405–8.

28. Ruston JC, Amin K, Karhouse N, et al. The vascularized medial femoral corticoperiosteal flap for thumb reconstruction. Plast Reconstr Surg Glob Open 2015;3(8):492.

29. Lin CH, Mardini S, Lin CH, et al. Osteoplastic thumb ray restoration with or without secondary toe transfer for reconstruction of opposable basic hand function. Plast Reconstr Surg 2008;121:1288–97.

30. Henry SL, Wei FC. Thumb reconstruction with toe transfer. J Hand Microsurg 2010;2(2):72–8.

31. Yim KK, Wei FC, Lin CH. A comparison between primary and secondary toe-to-hand transplantation. Plast Reconstr Surg 2004;114:107–12.

32. Woo SH, Lee GJ, Kim KC, et al. Immediate partial great toe transfer for the reconstruction of composite defects of the distal thumb. Plast Reconstr Surg 2006;117:1906–15.

Metacarpal-Like and Metacarpal Hand

Nidal Farhan ALDeek, MD, MSc[a], Yu-Te Lin, MD[a], Fu-Chan Wei, MD[b],*

KEYWORDS

- Toe-to-hand transfer • Metacarpal hand • Metacarpal-like hand • Second toe transfer
- Combined second and third toe transfer • Trimmed great toe transfer • Whole great toe transfer
- Tripod pinch

KEY POINTS

- Metacarpal-like and metacarpal hand are severe hand injuries that may benefit from microsurgical toe-to-hand transfer.
- The level of thumb and finger amputations, and the residual digits determine the types and subtypes of the metacarpal-like and metacarpal hand.
- The reconstruction of two adjacent fingers and opposable thumb is the core principle in the treatment of metacarpal-like and metacarpal hand injuries.
- In bilateral injuries, donor site selection and management after toe harvest is critical to avoid significant gait disturbances or daily activities restriction.

INTRODUCTION

Metacarpal hand is a severe debilitating hand injury. The term refers to the loss of all fingers proximal to the functional length with or without the thumb.[1] Although a clear consensus on what defines a functional length is lacking, it largely refers to the middle of the proximal phalanx. Given the injury, the hand lacks basic prehensile function, which is the ability to perform adequate opposition of the thumb to fingers.

The metacarpal-like hand, a novel term, refers to the amputation of all digits, fingers and thumb, proximal to the functional length, except in one or two digits, including the thumb. The term summarizes a diverse group of injuries that is in between proximal multiple finger amputation and metacarpal hand. Depending on the spared digits, that still maintain functional length, the hand may or may not still be able to provide proper basic prehensile function. For both injuries, classification and treatment algorithms are invaluable to guide surgeons in their endeavor to restore or enhance hand function and improve patient's quality of life.

METACARPAL HAND: CLASSIFICATION

In 1997, the senior author (F.-C.W.) proposed a classification for metacarpal hand injuries.[1] The intention was to provide a practical guideline for the classification and treatment of these injuries to achieve optimal function of the reconstructed hand while minimizing morbidity at the donor sites.

The metacarpal hand is divided into type I and type II. Type I includes the hand with amputations of all fingers proximal to the middle level of the proximal phalanx with either a normal thumb or a thumb that has been amputated distal to the interphalangeal joint.

Type II includes the hand with amputations of all fingers proximal to the middle portion of the proximal phalanx with amputation of the thumb

[a] Department of Plastic and Reconstructive Surgery, Chang Gung Memorial Hospital, Chang Gung Medical College, Chang Gung University, Taipei, Taiwan; [b] Department of Plastic and Reconstructive Surgery, Chang Gung Memorial Hospital, Chang Gung Medical College, Chang Gung University, 199 Tun-Hwa North Road, Taipei 10591, Taiwan
* Correspondence author.
E-mail address: fuchanwei@gmail.com

Hand Clin 32 (2016) 549–554
http://dx.doi.org/10.1016/j.hcl.2016.06.004
0749-0712/16/© 2016 Elsevier Inc. All rights reserved.

proximal to the interphalangeal joint. Type II is further subdivided into four subtypes depending on the level of thumb amputation, the presence of thenar musculature function, and the involvement of the basal joint.

METACARPAL-LIKE HAND: CLASSIFICATION

Although the metacarpal-like hand does not result in as much anatomic and functional deficits as the metacarpal hand, it could be similar in its functional impairment if core principles of reconstruction of metacarpal hand are to be adopted.

The metacarpal-like hand can also be divided into type I and type II. In type I, the thumb is either normal or amputated but with adequate length, at the level of interphalangeal joint, and function and one finger is normal or amputated but with adequate length.

In type II, the fingers are like type I, but the thumb is amputated proximal to the interphalangeal joint. Type II can be further subdivided into four subtypes following the same method used for type II metacarpal hand.

SURGICAL TREATMENT

Microsurgical toe-to-hand transfer remains the treatment of choice, although hand allotransplantation could be indicated for reconstruction of type IIb-c in the future when concerns about lifelong immunosuppressants side effects are largely resolved.

Toe-to-hand surgery takes into account the adequacy of soft tissue and bony stalk, involved digits, the level of amputation of each finger and thumb, and the presence or absence of thenar musculature. Unilaterality or bilaterality of the injury is also important in deciding on the optimal treatment plan, including donor site selection.[2] The surgery is done in a staged or one-stage arrangement depending on the level and type of injury.

Metacarpal Hand

A useful rule of thumb for metacarpal hand is to transplant a combined second and third toe (or combined fourth and fifth toe) or bilateral second toe (or bilateral third toe) for the reconstruction of two adjacent fingers in metacarpal hand type I and II, and to transfer a whole great toe, trimmed great toe (superior aesthetic results and equally safe in children),[3,4] or second toe for additional thumb reconstruction in metacarpal hand type II. When the thenar muscles or/and basal joint function is destroyed, finger reconstruction proceeds first followed by thumb reconstruction (staged reconstruction).

For patients with bilateral metacarpal hands type II, we recommend reconstructing the thumb of the dominant hand with a whole or trimmed left great toe and amputated fingers with either the left third and fourth toes or the right second and third toes or third and fourth toes, aiming at preserving right great toe for car driving. The two adjacent toes can be harvested in tandem or separated depending on the level of amputation (proximal or distal to the web space). The nondominant hand is reconstructed with individual left third and fourth toes or right second and third toes, one used for thumb and the other for one of the fingers.

Metacarpal-like Hand

A useful guideline is to transplant a whole great toe, trimmed great toe, or second toe for thumb reconstruction in type II and to reconstruct the amputated fingers in type I and II as follows. Single toe transfer should be used if the remaining finger is central (long or ring finger) or radial (index or long finger). Combined toe transfer is chosen if the remaining finger has poor function or stiff despite its adequate length. Double lesser toe is chosen to improve the condition of the remaining finger and reconstruct one more adjacent new finger. If the remaining finger is ulnar, basically the fifth finger is left, at least one toe should be transferred to allow hook function, but multiple toe transfer (double lesser toe or combined toe transfer) may grant more stability to hook function. Bilateral metacarpal-like hand type II is reconstructed in a manner similar to bilateral metacarpal hand type II with attention to the location of the remnant digits.

CASE 1

A 50-year-old man was diagnosed with metacarpal hand type I amputation. The patient received a pedicled groin flap with iliac crest bone graft first to replace the missing soft tissue and bony stalk. After uneventful healing of the pedicled flap, a combined second and third toe was transferred. After 25-year follow-up, good results can still be seen (**Fig. 1**).

CASE 2

A 44-year-old man was diagnosed with metacarpal hand type II amputation. The patient received staged reconstruction. At first, a pedicled groin flap with iliac bone graft was transferred, then a combined second and third toe was transplanted, and after 5 months the patient received second toe transfer for thumb reconstruction. Good results are shown after 24-year follow-up (**Fig. 2**).

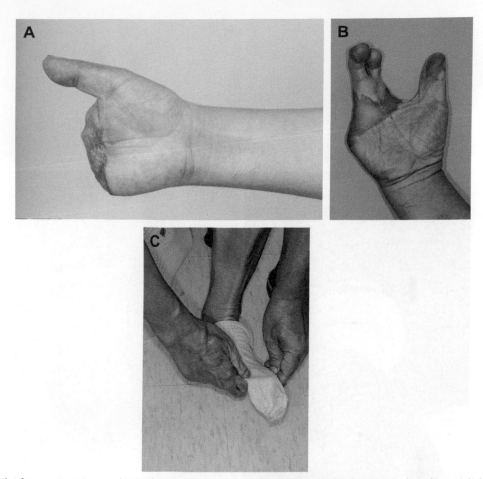

Fig. 1. (*A*) After amputation and initial care. (*B*) A combined second and third toe transfer after pedicled groin flap with iliac bone graft. (*C*) Effective use of the reconstructed hand in daily activity is shown.

CASE 3

A 44-year-old man was diagnosed with metacarpal hand type II amputation. The patient received staged reconstruction. At first, a pedicled groin flap with iliac bone graft was transferred, then a combined second and third toe was transplanted, and after 5 months the patient received second toe transfer for thumb reconstruction. Good results are shown after 24-year follow-up (**Fig. 3**).

DISCUSSION

Microsurgical toe transfers have been used successfully for the reconstruction of metacarpal hand injuries.[1,2,5–10] The metacarpal-like hand injuries may share common features with the metacarpal hand and could, therefore, benefit from the same surgical approach.

Several principles must be followed when dealing with the metacarpal and metacarpal-like

hand injuries to optimize functional outcomes. Planning for toe-to-hand surgery should start during the initial evaluation and treatment at emergency setting. The surgeon must preserve the length of bone, tendons, and neurovascular bundles whenever possible,[11] and preserve intact joint surfaces.

The surgeon should also assess the adequacy of the soft tissue and the length of residual metacarpus (bony stalk), and then replace missing coverage and/or bone avoiding local tissue and free flap, preserving the recipient vessels for microsurgical transplantation of toes. The pedicled groin flap alone or with inclusion of iliac crest is a good choice for secondary toe-to-hand transfer, because it provides ample tissue and honors the goal of tissue preservation.

In metacarpal-like and metacarpal hand type II, the first metacarpus could be short if the remaining length of the metacarpal bone is functionally inadequate. Lengthening is important to avoid harvesting a long great toe, which usually

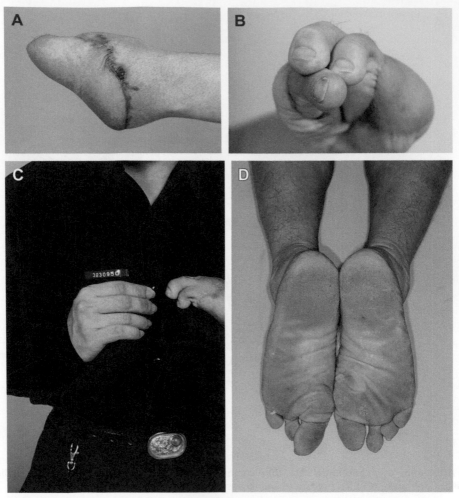

Fig. 2. (*A*) Pedicled groin flap with iliac bone graft. (*B*) After combined second and third toe transfer and second toe transfer, a stable tripod pinch is noted. (*C*) Effective use of the reconstructed hand in daily activity. (*D*) No web space widening, scissoring, or callus formation.

results in increased morbidity at the donor site. Several techniques are available to overcome a short first metacarpal bone, including bone lengthening using distraction osteogenesis or free nonvascularized bone graft, and use of second toe transfer instead of great toe transfer. In addition, when the thenar musculature is involved in metacarpal-like and metacarpal hand (type IIC), we prefer to stage the reconstruction.

The suggested surgical algorithms aim at reconstructing two adjacent fingers and thumb to restore tripod pinch, lateral stability, a stable hook grip, and a wider span for grasping larger objects.[6–8,12]

Combined second and third or third and fourth toe transfers are chosen if the amputations are proximal enough so that a syndactylous appearance is avoided,[9,10,13] and single toe transfers

are performed when the amputations are distal to the web space.[14,15] The digits to be reconstructed are chosen based on the patient's vocational needs. The ulnar digits are reconstructed when a strong grip is desired, and the radial digits are reconstructed when fine manipulation is the goal.

Toe harvest starts with pedicle identification at the web space followed by retrograde dissection.[6,16] One artery and one vein are enough except in combined second and third toe; a second artery is prepared and used when needed.[17] Bilateral injuries are managed using the same principles as for unilateral injuries, with some modifications in donor site selection. Because at least four to five toes are required for the complete reconstruction, emphasis is placed on minimizing gait disturbances. Therefore, in the most severe cases (bilateral type II), we aim at achieving a

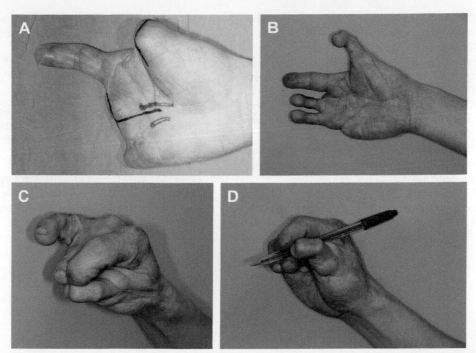

Fig. 3. (*A*) The hand after injury; the index was spared with adequate functional length. (*B*) The second toe for thumb reconstruction in the functional position. (*C*) Tripod pinch involving the native index. (*D*) Good use of small objects, such as a pen, based on effective tripod pinch.

tripod pinch in the dominant hand and compromise with pulp-to-pulp pinch in the nondominant hand. When one of the hands is type I, a tripod pinch is achieved in both hands without additional donor site morbidity.

Donor site morbidity is higher when the great toe is harvested followed by the combined second and third toe followed by the second toe; therefore, we prefer to leave behind at least the great toe and two other toes (usually the fourth and fifth toes) in the right foot and the second and fifth toes in the left foot. The choice of toes is based on what is required to maintain balance during stationary positioning and ambulation and takes into consideration the importance of the right foot in daily activities, such as driving.[2]

SUMMARY

The metacarpal-like and metacarpal hands can be reconstructed with multiple toe transfers. Our approach of reconstructing opposable digits, preferably tripod pinch rather than pulp-to-pulp or pulp-to-side pinch, has better functional results. With this concept and approach, hands can be reconstructed to become useful and functional despite the devastating presentation of the initial injury.

REFERENCES

1. Wei FC, El-Gammal TA, Lin CH, et al. Metacarpal hand: classification and guidelines for microsurgical reconstruction with toe transfers. Plast Reconstr Surg 1997;99:122.
2. Wei FC, Lutz BS, Cheng SL, et al. Reconstruction of bilateral metacarpal hands with multiple-toe transplantations. Plast Reconstr Surg 1999;104:1698.
3. Mardini S, Wei FC. Unilateral and bilateral metacarpal hand injuries: classification and treatment guidelines. Plast Reconstr Surg 2004;113(6):1756–9.
4. Wei FC, Chen HC, Chuang CC, et al. Reconstruction of the thumb with a trimmed toe transfer technique. Plast Reconstr Surg 1988;82:506.
5. Tan BK, Wei FC, Lutz BS, et al. Strategies in multiple toe transplantation for bilateral type II metacarpal hand reconstruction. Hand Clin 1999;15:607.
6. Wei FC, Colony LH. Microsurgical reconstruction of opposable digits in mutilating hand injuries. Clin Plast Surg 1989;16:491.
7. Wei FC, Coessens B, Ganos D. Multiple microsurgical toe-to-hand transfer in the reconstruction of the severely mutilated hand: a series of fifty-nine cases. Ann Chir Main Memb Super 1992;11:177.
8. Tsai TM, Jupiter JB, Wolff TW, et al. Reconstruction of severe transmetacarpal mutilating hand injuries by combined second and third toe transfer. J Hand Surg Am 1981;6:319.

9. Tan BK, Wei FC, Chang KJ, et al. Combined third and fourth toe transplantation. Hand Clin 1999;15:589.

10. Wei FC, Strauch RJ, Chen HC, et al. Reconstruction of four damaged or destroyed ipsilateral fingers with free toe-to-hand transplantations. Plast Reconstr Surg 1994;93:608.

11. Wei FC. Tissue preservation in hand injury: the first step to toe-to-hand transplantation. Plast Reconstr Surg 1998;102:2497.

12. Wei FC, Chen HC, Chuang CC, et al. Simultaneous multiple toe transfers in hand reconstruction. Plast Reconstr Surg 1988;81:366.

13. Wei FC, Colony LH, Chen HC, et al. Combined second and third toe transfer. Plast Reconstr Surg 1989; 84:651.

14. Lutz BS, Wei FC. Basic principles on toe-to-hand transplantation. Chang Gung Med J 2002;25:568.

15. Wei FC, Silverman RT, Hsu WM. Retrograde dissection of the vascular pedicle in toe harvest. Plast Reconstr Surg 1995;96:1211.

16. Wei FC, Mardini S. Re-evaluation of the technique of toe-to-hand transfer for traumatic digital amputations in children and adolescents. Plast Reconstr Surg 2003;112:1870.

17. Cheng MH, Wei FC, Santamaria E, et al. Single versus double arterial anastomoses in combined second- and third-toe transplantation. Plast Reconstr Surg 1998;102(7):2408–12 [discussion: 2413].

Secondary Interventions for Mutilating Hand Injuries

Anthony Foo, MD*, Sandeep J. Sebastin, MD

KEYWORDS

- Mutilating hand injures • Mangled hand • Hand reconstruction • Secondary reconstruction

KEY POINTS

- Secondary procedures are frequently required to improve function of reconstructed mutilated hands.
- They should be tailored to patients' unique vocational, functional, and recreational requirements.
- Secondary procedures may be broadly divided into obligatory procedures and discretionary procedures.
- Obligatory procedures refer to interventions done to complete staged reconstructions or address complications arising from primary procedures.
- Discretionary procedures refer to interventions done to improve function or appearance of the hand. They should only be undertaken when the patient has been psychologically and physiologically optimized.

INTRODUCTION

Successful restoration of good hand function at the primary admission for a mutilating hand injury is uncommon. In most cases, primary treatment aims to salvage available functional units with staged reconstruction in mind.[1–3] The indications for secondary interventions (**Table 1**) may be broadly divided into obligatory and discretionary procedures. Obligatory procedures are required to complete staged reconstructions and address complications. These interventions are time-sensitive and are undertaken based on timeline of tissue healing. Discretionary procedures, however, are undertaken to improve function and/or enhance appearance of the reconstructed hand. Outcomes of these procedures depend largely on patient expectation and motivation. It is therefore important to psychologically and physiologically optimize patients before considering discretionary procedures.

OBLIGATORY SURGICAL PROCEDURES
Completion of Staged Primary Procedures

Primary reconstruction in mutilating injuries is aimed at providing expedient skeletal stabilization, microvascular anastomosis, repositioning of functional units, and soft tissue cover of critical defects. In most situations, this entails use of external fixators, interosseous wiring, and flap coverage. As patients recover, some of the provisional measures can be modified for comfort and mobility.

Soft tissue procedures

Large soft tissue defects are usually covered with a combination of flap and skin graft. Critical defects exposing neurovascular structures, webspaces, and joints are best covered with flap, whereas other areas may be covered with skin graft (**Fig. 1**). Tissue quality of noncritical regions may be improved with the use of negative pressure wound therapy and

Department of Hand & Reconstructive Microsurgery, National University Health System, 1E Kent Ridge Road, Singapore 119228, Singapore
* Corresponding author.
E-mail address: anthony_foo@nuhs.edu.sg

Hand Clin 32 (2016) 555–567
http://dx.doi.org/10.1016/j.hcl.2016.07.006
0749-0712/16/© 2016 Elsevier Inc. All rights reserved.

Table 1
Indications for secondary reconstruction in mutilated hands

		Soft Tissue Procedures	Bone and Joint Procedures
Obligatory procedures	Complete staged procedures	Skin grafting/flap division Tendon grafting Nerve grafting	Conversion of ex-fix Bone grafting Arthrodesis
	Address complications	Infection Scar contracture and adhesions Neuropathic pain and neuroma	Osteomyelitis Joint stiffness Nonunion and malunion
Discretionary procedures	Augment function	Tendon transfer Toe transfer Amputation Hand transplant	
	Enhance appearance	Flap debulking Scar revision Tissue expansion Prosthesis	

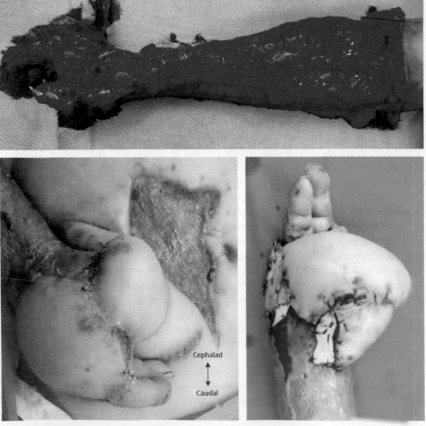

Cephalad

Caudal

Fig. 1. Defect initially covered with skin graft can be excised and resurfaced with groin flap in preparation for second stage procedure. (*Courtesy of* Dr A. Lahiri, MD, Department of Hand & Reconstructive Microsurgery, National University Health System, Singapore.)

engineered dermal matrices before skin grafting.[4,5] Granulation tissue formed with negative pressure wound therapy improves contour for skin graft adhesion, whereas engineered matrices allow formation of neodermis that lessens secondary skin graft contracture. Infrequently, skin grafting is required to resurface the residual defects following debridement of compromised flaps.

Pedicled groin or abdominal flaps are reliable options that can provide coverage for large defects. They have the added advantage of preserving vessels in the limb for future microvascular reconstruction. Between 2 and 3 weeks, a delay process is initiated in preparation for flap division by application of mechanical devices, such as bowel clamps and ligatures, or strategic delay by surgical incisions. After division, the edges of the flaps are trimmed and contoured to blend into the overall appearance of the hand.

Multiple tendon loss and unsuitable wound bed are indications for two-stage tendon reconstruction with silastic rods and coverage with fasciocutaneous flap to facilitate interval access for tendon grafting.[6] During this time, passive mobilization is essential to prevent stiffness of the affects joints and prevent edema.

Nerves are invariably injured and there may be multiple nerve involvement with nerve gaps following debridement. Primary nerve repair may not be carried out because of unfavorable wound conditions, or questionable survival of target muscles. If secondary nerve grafting is planned, nerve ends can be tagged with 5/0 polypropylene sutures and placed subcutaneously to facilitate retrieval at the next procedure.[7] Sensory nerve repair or grafting offers reasonable chance of restoring sensation of the injured digits, whereas motor nerve repair should be performed after assessing the muscles. Traumatized intrinsic muscles rarely regain meaningful function. Nerve grafts, particularly autologous, are therefore best reserved for sensory reconstruction.[8] Motor nerve repair for intrinsic muscles of the hand is unpredictable,[9,10] particularly when intrinsic muscles are injured; therefore early tendon transfers or finger joint fusions may be considered for reconstructing intrinsic hand function.

Bone and joint procedures

Initial skeletal stabilization with external fixator or interosseous wiring may be performed because of limited soft tissue cover or uncertain viability of amputated parts. As patients' physiology and local soft tissue condition stabilize, hardware internalization is advantageous to facilitate rehabilitation. Fractures through phalanges and metacarpals are often adequately stabilized with wires and usually do not require internal fixation. However, injuries through the carpus or the distal radius and ulna benefit from conversion from spanning fixators to internal fixation with plates and screws. This may be performed in tandem with skin grafting or flap cover, planned with future procedures in mind, such as bone or tendon reconstruction.

Bone loss is common in severe crush injuries and defects that are not suitable for shortening or primary bone grafting may be filled with bone cement and stabilized with an external fixator. In sufficiently vascularized wounds, a pseudomembrane forms around the cement spacer, providing a favorable condition for secondary bone grafting with cancellous chips.[11] The formation of the pseudomembrane takes approximately 6 weeks at which point the second stage can be done. This involves elevation of tissue flaps, cement spacer extrication, packing of cancellous chips into the defect without disrupting the pseudomembrane, and internal fixation. The elevation of fasciocutaneous flaps is easier compared with muscle flaps and this may be a consideration in choice of flap coverage. The volume of bone graft required determines the donor site. Arbitrarily, the distal radius of a young adult reliably provides up to 2 mL (measured on a 5-mL syringe) of cancellous chips, whereas the iliac crest is more reliable for larger volumes (more than 2 mL) and older adults.[12]

Complications Resulting from Primary Reconstruction

The main physiologic changes at the zone of injury are heightened inflammatory response and tissue hypoxia. Heightened inflammatory responses predispose adhesion formation and scar contraction, leading to pain, stiffness, and deformity. Retained microscopic foreign body or foci of nonviable tissue can act as a nidus for infection. Despite successful microvascular salvage, blood supply to tissues, such as bone, periosteum, and tendon, can be tenuous, leaving these tissues at risk of nonunion or rupture of repair. These complications are broadly divided into soft tissue and bone related groups.

Soft tissue complications

These complications include infection, adhesions, scar contracture, and neuropathic pain.

Infection

Soft tissue infections range from localized focal abscesses to widespread disseminated infection and these are strong indications for surgical intervention. Infection can arise from retained foreign material, nonviable tissue, and colonization at the primary treatment. Radiolucent contaminants and toxic chemical compounds (acid, alkali, alcohol, flame retardant, and so forth) are difficult to identity and may result in delayed tissue necrosis. Introduction of sutures and implants may further contribute to tissue trauma and escalate the risk of infection in severely traumatized wounds.

The principle of managing infection is to distinguish between deep infections arising from devitalized tissue, sequestrum, and foreign material from those arising from surface colonization. The former may manifest with discharging sinuses, and tenderness with or without surface cellulitis. Diagnosis is mainly clinical. Adjuncts, such as differential blood counts, inflammatory markers, and imaging, may be helpful. From the surgical perspective, a tumorlike approach to debridement must be undertaken with caution and attention to potentially distorted positions of neurovascular structures and flap pedicles.[13] These structures are difficult to identify in the field of injury. Therefore, extensile incisions are recommended to facilitate identification in normal anatomy before proceeding into the zone of trauma.

Scar contracture

Scar contraction is mediated by myofibroblasts during the remodeling phase of tissue healing and its primary effects are reduction in mobility of mobile tissues (skin, tendon, nerve, and joints).[14,15] Once primary wound healing takes place, emollients and silicone sheets should be judiciously applied to maintain skin hydration and suppleness, in tandem with pressure garments and splints. Dry skin causes itch, which lends itself to excoriation and fissuring that eventually limits mobilization and leads to noncompliance to splinting.

Edema needs to be treated early. Left unchecked, edema fluid that is mobile and reducible in its early state develops a brawny consistency that does not reduce with compression.[16] Skin changes in the latter state are usually permanent with little chance of reversal. Hence, edema management and compression garment must be instituted as soon as possible to avert this unfavorable state.

Linear scars across joints and webspaces limit joint mobility and web span. Scars that fail to soften with conservative measures are considered for Z-plasty lengthening and use of dermal substitutes or full-thickness skin graft. Split-thickness skin grafts are best avoided for palmar and webspace regions because of its propensity for secondary contracture. Scars in the palm may contract centripetally, drawing radial and ulnar digits toward each other, limiting grasp span and digitopalmar grip. Scar excision followed by fasciocutaneous flap interposition may be required to prevent future contracture and improve hand function.

Neuropathic pain and neuroma

The sequelae of neurapraxic and axonometic injuries are epineurial scarring and formation of neuroma in continuity.[17,18] Resultant motor and/or sensory deficits may improve spontaneously or require surgical intervention.[19–21] Serial examinations over 3 to 6 months with monofilament sensory mapping and Tinel percussion test provides a general idea of nerve recovery and useful milestones for surgical intervention. Lack of improvement after an observation period of 6 months is an arbitrary time-frame for intervention for pain or paresthesia relief. The role of motor reconstruction in the mutilated hand is limited by the lack of functional muscle units. At 6 months, tissues in the zone of injury should have equilibrated and surgical intervention is manageable.[22]

In most cases, nerves with diameter of less than 2 mm are difficult to identify in a traumatized field and microscope magnification is recommended. The surgeon should identify three key features during nerve exploration: (1) surrounding scar tissue, (2) epineurium, and (3) overall nerve morphology. Scar release without neurolysis would suffice if the epineurium of the nerve exhibits minimal or focal thickening corresponding to scar bands, whereas neurolysis is indicated if there were segmental thickening and narrowing of the nerve. Segmental narrowing and hourglass-shaped nerves may indicate presence of lesion in continuity and neurolysis allows internal examination of the nerve for intact fascicles.[23,24] Stretched-out fascicles without clearly identifiable neural elements are excised and replaced with autografts or allografts, with or without conduit. The outcome of neurolysis and nerve grafting is fairly variable, and it is best to manage patients' expectations from the outset.[25] One hopes for the best while expecting the worst.

Neuromas may develop from transected nerve ends, causing exquisite contact pain and tenderness that severely limits activities of daily living. Nerve repair or grafting may be considered if distal end of the nerve is identifiable, whereas end neuromas without distal stump may be buried within muscle or bone to avoid further symptomatic nerve sprouts.[26,27] Another possibility is to perform centrocentral union type coaptation between cut ends of nerves or looping it onto itself to mitigate the risk of neuroma formation.[28] A multitude of technique has been reported with satisfactory but unpredictable outcomes.[26]

Bone and joint complications

These complications include osteomyelitis, joint stiffness, malunion, and nonunion.

Osteomyelitis

The high-energy trauma causes impaction of foreign material, such as gravel or soil particles, deep into the medullary canal that evades detection. Periosteal stripping and physical insult of hardware insertion during fracture fixation further embarrasses blood supply to bone and periosteum, setting the stage for osteonecrosis and osteomyelitis. Acute osteomyelitis may present with pain and swelling and is best treated expediently with excision of sequestrum, drainage of pus, coverage with vascular tissue, and parenteral antibiotics.[29,30] Hardware removal is indicated only if the screw holes are involved, rather than routinely, to avert the situation of concurrent instability and infection. Conversion to external fixator is often not practical and thermal damage from insertion of fixator pins can be considerable, given the size and scale of hand bones. Principles that apply to a tibia do not necessarily hold true for non-weight-bearing metacarpals and phalanges. In the presence of extensive bone involvement, salvage procedures and amputation should be discussed. Successful bone salvage does not always imply good functional outcome and ray amputation may return patients to function earlier (**Fig. 2**).

Inadequately treated osteomyelitis may lead to chronic infection that is difficult to eradicate.[31–33] Methicillin-resistant *Staphylococcus aureus* infection can assume latent stages with infrequent

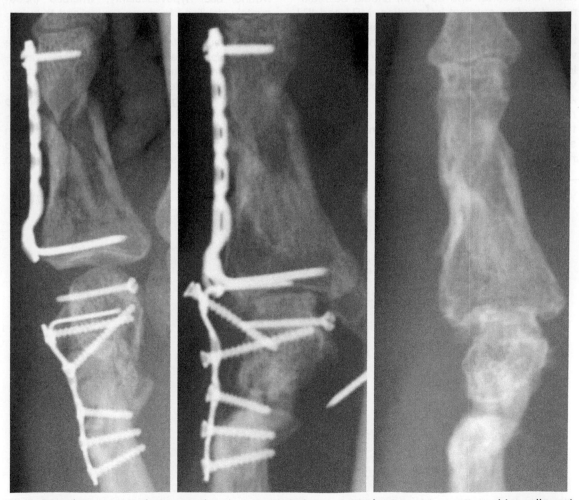

Fig. 2. Severely comminuted metacarpal neck reconstructed with cortical struts and cancellous chips collapsed caused by local infection, osteonecrosis, and graft resorption. Although successfully salvaged, there was little motion of the small finger.

exacerbation despite aggressive treatment. Biofilm formation and bony lacunae provide sanctuary sites for microbial colonization, necessitating radical bone excision to achieve complete eradication. However, the impact of radical surgery needs to be weighed against manifestations of chronic osteomyelitis before embarking on the arduous reconstructive journey that could last for months.

Joint stiffness

Edema, pain, and inadequate therapy lead to poor hand position and joint stiffness. Interphalangeal joints (IPJ) followed by metacarpophalangeal joints (MPJ) are the most vulnerable. Both joints rely on intrinsic muscles for its mobility and the constrained ginglymoid architecture of the former compounds the problem of stiffness.[34,35] Analgesics, anti-inflammatory medications, and passive stretching with therapy modalities (massage, heat, ultrasound, and so forth) should be maximized before surgical intervention. MPJ and IPJ releases are indicated in the presence of functioning intrinsic muscles and should be undertaken with caution if the interossei are damaged.[36] The long-term results of IPJ release are unpredictable, whereas MPJ release offers better outcomes.[37,38] An intrinsic minus hand with stiff joints poorly responsive to therapy should be evaluated for the possibility of improving position with IPJ fusions, given the poor results of contracture release.

Malunion

The severity of tissue distortion and loss in these injuries may complicate judgment and assessment during the initial treatment. Digit position or length following heterotopic replantation or pollicization may not satisfy patients' activity requirements and surgery may be indicated to improve hand function. Thumb ray lengthening is helpful to increase grasp span and reach of opposition to the ulnar digit. In its anatomic positions, the thumb opposes the small finger at a tangent, in a pincer manner. Although this is sufficient for manipulation of medium to large objects, patients wishing to manipulate fine objects with these digits may be offered rotation osteotomy of the small finger metacarpal to alter the direction of pulp-to-pulp contact between the thumb and little finger (**Fig. 3**).

Nonunion

Fracture nonunion may be atrophic because of wound bed hypovascularity, whereas inadequately stabilized fractures are inclined to hypertrophic nonunion. Atrophic nonunion is treated by biologic augmentation with vascularized bone graft or flap transfer is indicated to improve vascularity of the fracture site, in addition to stable osteosynthesis. Regional carpal-arch-based vascularized bone grafts are often not available because of vessel damage, hence free osteocutaneous or osteomyocutaneous flap options from medial femoral condyle, fibula, iliac crest, and so forth may be considered. Hypertrophic nonunion

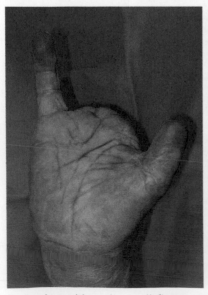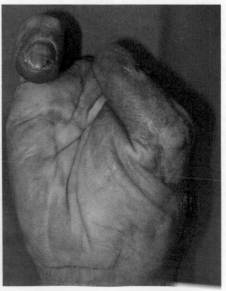

Fig. 3. In its anatomic position, the small finger and thumb oppose diagonally. A shortened thumb may be considered for lengthening or toe transfer to improve pincer grip mechanism. A rotation osteotomy of the fifth metacarpus is an alternative consideration to improve precision of the pinch.

is caused by inadequate stability for mineralization of fracture callous and the principles of treatment are excision of fibrous callous to obtain bone contact between fracture ends. Plates and screws are more rigid as compared with wires or external fixators and whenever possible the former is the construct of choice in treatment of nonunion. Autologous cancellous bone chips may be used to bridge small gaps following revision fixation.

DISCRETIONARY SURGICAL PROCEDURES

These procedures are undertaken to augment function or improve appearance of the reconstructed hand. These procedures are patient dependent and not time dependent. The most important aspect of discretionary procedures is to determine patient suitability for these procedures. The patient must be psychologically and physiologically optimized for the procedure and local tissue condition should have equilibrated before embarking on discretionary surgical procedures.

Psychological Assessment

Physical and psychological pain often coexist and it is vital to distinguish one from the other. Psychological optimization is as important as surgical intervention to relieve pain. Patient assessment following primary reconstruction begins with psychological profiling to determine social and vocational coping mechanisms.[39] Characteristics of a well-adjusted patient include good self-grooming and hygiene, awareness and acceptance of physical limitation with lifestyle and workplace activity modification and neutral to positive outlook on life after injury. Red flags of poor adjustment include neglect of injured hand and personal grooming, reference to the injured hand as third party, overwhelming focus on the injury, anger with circumstances leading to injury, and negative outlook on life with signs suggestive of potential for self-harm or suicide.[40,41] The most common cause is workplace trauma and it afflicts blue collar workers with limited financial means. Hence, financial concerns for self and their families weigh heavily in decision making. Psychiatric assessment and/or social worker involvement early in the recovery period is helpful to aid psychosocial adaptation and reintegration into society. Secondary surgical intervention in the latter group is fraught with difficulties that may be beyond the surgeon's control, and should be undertaken with caution. A strong indication for intervention is infection that threatens the hand or life. Discretionary procedures for functional refinement are contraindicated for patients still undergoing psychological adjustment.

The mainstay of secondary interventions for psychologically adjusting patients is medications, physical therapy, and psychotherapy. Severe physical trauma and its treatment leave massive psychological footprints.[39,40] Pain is a major issue and it originates from inflammation and tissue healing, nerve injury, and cortical psychic pain. A cocktail of analgesics, anti-inflammatory drugs (nonsteroidal anti-inflammatory, cyclooxygenase-2), neuroleptics, antidepressants, and anticonvulsants, with or without psychological counseling, is often required. Early review by pain specialists is helpful, and if signs of depression or posttraumatic stress disorder are present, psychiatry review is helpful. Apart from pain, enquiry about patients' sleep pattern and observation for signs of insomnia or hypersomnolence, blood shot eyes, or poor attention span may elucidate unresolved issues. A short course (5–10 days) of benzodiazepine to facilitate sleep could completely transform a patient for the following review.

Psychological recovery is uncertain and often confounded by other circumstances, such as limited social support, financial means, and communication barrier with health care providers caused by cultural differences. Hence, the objectives of nonsurgical secondary treatment are psychological and social support, expedited rehabilitation, and payout of workers' injury compensation. Interpreters are an invaluable resource in establishing rapport with patients of diverse cultural backgrounds to foster understanding of their motivations and challenges and setting rehabilitation goals. An additional consideration is the vulnerability of these patients to opportunistic lawyers, legal representatives and interest group lobbyists that often delay the final assessment for settlement of injury compensation. Licensed migrant workers are often subjected to employment permit conditions and face repatriation if their injury disability exceeds a predetermined percentage.

Functional Assessment

Physical assessment of psychologically adjusted patients begins with morphologic assessment of the reconstructed extremity. It is imperative to establish patients' understanding of the "ideal beautiful normal" and their appreciation of the baseline function.[42,43] Function does not always follow form and vice versa in hand reconstruction. An unsightly hand with a bulky flap and functional thumb may work better than an "acceptable hand" with a thumb and three digits. The next factor to consider in designing intervention is the availability of functioning intrinsic muscle units. Hands devoid of intrinsic musculature are characterized by intrinsic minus posture with stiff joints and function primarily as the assist hand. Finger reanimation is unrealistic and the priority is therefore aimed at wrist joint mobility or stability, improving sensation of the hand, pain alleviation, and correction of gross deformities.

The final consideration before surgical intervention is pain and tissue equilibrium state.[22] Pain management is important to facilitate therapy and the approach is similar to the previously discussed method. Tissue healing transits from inflammatory to remodeling in the weeks and months following trauma, achieving an equilibrated stated where signs of inflammation, such as tenderness, edema and erythema resolve. Salmon pink or purplish, raised, painful scars indicate ongoing inflammatory and remodeling processes. Tissues in this state are unsuitable for elective intervention because of the risk of inducing further inflammation and dissection through friable tissue in transition state is difficult. This phase is reported to last between 3 and 6 months and only time-sensitive obligatory procedures are considered. Reconstruction to augment function is best undertaken after tissue equilibrium is achieved. Interim measures that may expedite the transition include edema control by compressive garments, splinting, active-passive mobilization, and topical/systemic anti-inflammatory medications.

Discretionary Procedures to Augment Function

Tendon transfers

The permutation and choice of tendon transfer is determined by the extent of injury and the resultant deficits.[44,45] Tendon transfer and grafting may be part of a primary procedure or indicated later to strengthen remaining musculotendinous units that are weak. Opponensplasty-type transfers may be performed to strengthen the thumb ray grasp, whereas multislip flexor sublimis transfer can partially restore function of damaged intrinsic muscles. Further refinements include calibration of grasp by side-to-side tenodesis of flexor profundus slips or functional gracilis transfer in situations where the extrinsic muscles are severely damaged.[44]

Toe transfers

Toe transfer is an integral part of functional refinement of the mutilated hand. Primary indications for toe transfer are thumb loss and reconstruction of an ulnar post for pincer grip. The thumb ray is offset from the hand, providing exceptional mobility and versatility, accounting for nearly 50% of total function of the hand. Hentz proposed a practical classification that guides treatment of thumb ray loss.[43] Moderate functional impairment is expected with injuries around the IPJ of the thumb and can be improved with thumb lengthening, or partial toe transfers. The toe transfer is indicated for thumb loss between the MPJ and the carpometacarpal joint and pollicization considered when the thumb loss includes the carpometacarpal joint. The next priority following reconstruction of the thumb post is to reconstitute an opposition post for pinch and grip. A toe positioned along the fourth or fifth rays provides wide hand span at the cost of precision and strength. A wide hand span is advantageous to patients whose primary activity with the injured hand is handling medium to large objects. Toes positioned at the second or third rays provide strength and precision while forgoing hand span (**Fig. 4**). Double toe transfers to the intermediate rays provide strong and precise chuck pinch suitable for activities that demand these grip attributes.[45,46] Although it is possible to reconstruct all five digits with toe transfers, this approach is not often undertaken because the additional functional gain probably does not outweigh the morbidity of doing so. A special consideration for hands amputated at the level of the wrist is the Vilkki procedure, where a toe is transferred to the distal forearm for pinch reconstruction in patients with amputated stumps.[47]

Amputation

Another area of functional improvement is the assessment of the function of reconstructed digits. Stiff, nonfunctional fingers may impede the contact between the thumb and the ulnar digits. In select cases, shortening of the afflicted segments of the digit may be discussed. Ray amputation is not favored because this narrows the span of the hand, thereby limiting their repertoire of possible activities.

Hand transplant

Hand transplant represents the frontier of composite tissue allotransplantation, and should be kept in mind as an option in patients with mangled stumps without suitable tissue for toe transfers, or patients seeking functional improvement without resorting to toe transfer. The ethical barrier to hand transplantation is the feasibility of lifelong immunosuppression for a functional rather than life-saving procedure and the yet unresolved risks of immunosuppression.[48]

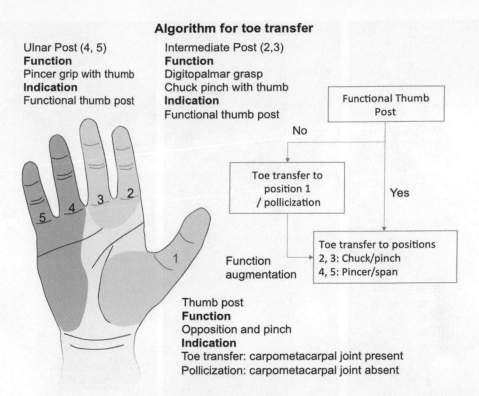

Algorithm for toe transfer

Ulnar Post (4, 5)
Function
Pincer grip with thumb
Indication
Functional thumb post

Intermediate Post (2,3)
Function
Digitopalmar grasp
Chuck pinch with thumb
Indication
Functional thumb post

Functional Thumb Post

No

Toe transfer to position 1 / pollicization

Yes

Function augmentation

Toe transfer to positions 2, 3: Chuck/pinch 4, 5: Pincer/span

Thumb post
Function
Opposition and pinch
Indication
Toe transfer: carpometacarpal joint present
Pollicization: carpometacarpal joint absent

Fig. 4. Toe transfers are planned based on the geographical deficit. A thumb post is the basic requirement, augmented by another toe along the ulnar or intermediate posts, for span or strength, respectively.

Discretionary Procedures to Improve Appearance

Flap debulking

A slightly oversized flap may be designed to provide soft tissue cover or prepare the traumatized region in anticipation of toe transfer or osteoplastic thumb reconstruction. In some instances, the bulk of the flap may obstruct digit opposition and movement, requiring debulking or partial excision to improve function and appearance. This is achieved by liposuction techniques or partial excision to achieve desired shape and thickness. Thick fat pads of fasciocutaneous flaps impede fine object manipulation and are improved by thinning and tightening the flap (**Fig. 5**).

Scar/skin graft revision and tissue expansion

Skin grafted areas often become hyperpigmented especially in nonwhite populations. In addition, these areas are often depressed in comparison with the surrounding skin because of a lack of dermal support and subcutaneous fat. A serial excision of the skin grafted areas can lead to a significant improvement of the appearance. Similarly, wide depressed scars are improved by de-epithelizing the scar and suturing the adjoining skin flaps over the de-epithelized scar using subcuticular nonabsorbable sutures. This addresses the depressed scar and helps in keeping the scar narrow. The technique of subcision can be considered in narrow depressed scars. Other options include the use of dermal fillers and fat grafts. Finally, the use of tissue expanders may be considered. It is infrequently used in the upper limb because of anatomic constraints, but may be considered if there were available adjacent expandable skin.[49,50]

Prosthesis

Short digits with inadequate reach may be considered for prosthesis. The overall aesthetic is greatly improved with prosthesis. Commercially available prosthesis offers highly realistic skin tones and subtle docking interfaces (**Fig. 6**). Although short-term patient acceptance is excellent, patients may be discouraged in the longer term because of inconvenience and costs of replacement. Osseointegrated implants show promising results to improve aesthetics and function.[51,52] The advantage of stability from bone docking is weighed against the challenge of obtaining a long-term seal at the soft tissue–implant interface (**Fig. 7**).

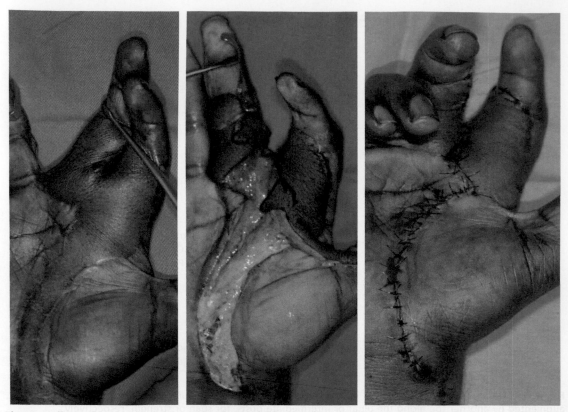

Fig. 5. Bulbous flap interposed between thumb, index, and middle fingers partially excised and trimmed to deepen second web space and thenar crease to improve dexterity of radial digits.

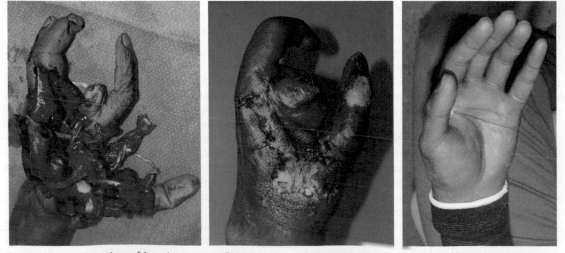

Fig. 6. Severe distortion of hand structures by grenade explosion required pollicization and skin grafting, Secondary procedures were performed to contour and span for prosthesis fit. (*Courtesy of* Mark Puhaindran, MD, Singapore.)

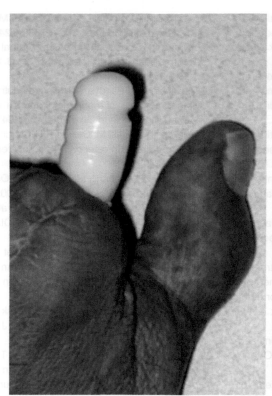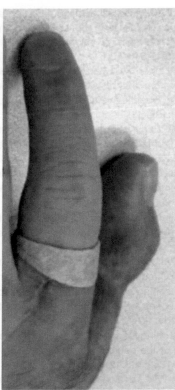

Fig. 7. Osseointegration provides a firm mechanical anchor in digits with inadequate stump for standard socket fit prosthesis. The docking mechanism provides a secure fit for various prosthesis options. (*Courtesy of* Mr Michael Leow, M.Sc., Prosthetic Lab, Department of Hand & Reconstructive Microsurgery, National University Health System, Singapore.)

SUMMARY

Secondary intervention for mutilated hand is a complex undertaking, with varied goals and individual specific outcomes. Surgeons' and patients' ability to continuously improvise and adapt the remaining functional units of the hand to the travails of life is paramount to achieving long-term satisfaction from reconstruction of the mutilated hand.

REFERENCES

1. Del Pinal F. Severe mutilating injuries to the hand: guidelines for organizing the chaos. J Plast Reconstr Aesthet Surg 2006;60:816–27.
2. Chong AK. Principles in management of a mangled hand. Indian J Plast Surg 2011;44:219–26.
3. Russell RC, Bueno RA, Wu TTY. Secondary procedures following mutilating hand injuries. Hand Clin 2003;19:149–63.
4. Webster J, Scuffham P, Satnkiewicz M, et al. Negative pressure wound therapy for skin grafts and surgical wounds healing by primary intention. Cochrane Database Syst Rev 2014;(10):CD009261.
5. Milcheski DA, Chang AA, Lobato RC, et al. Coverage of deep cutaneous wounds using dermal template in combination with negative pressure therapy and subsequent skin graft. Plast Reconstr Surg Glob Open 2014;2:e170.
6. Schneider LH. Staged flexor tendon reconstruction using the method of Hunter. Clin Orthop Relat Res 1982;171:164–71.
7. Sabapathy SR, Venkatramani H, Bharathi RR, et al. Technical considerations and functional outcome of 22 major replantations (The BSSH Douglas Lamb Lecture, 2005). J Hand Surg Eur Vol 2007;32(5):488–501.
8. Chevrollier J, Pedetour B, Dap F, et al. Evaluation of emergency nerve grafting for proper palmar digital nerve defects: a retrospective single centre study. Orthop Traumatol Surg Res 2014;100:605–10.
9. Vastamaki M, Kallio PK, Solonen KA. The results of secondary microsurgical repair of ulnar nerve injury. J Hand Surg 1993;18B:323–6.
10. Kayo H, Minami A, Kobayashi M, et al. Functional results of low median and ulnar nerve repair with intraneural fascicular dissection and electrical fascicular orientation. J Hand Surg 1998;23A:471–82.

Challenges Posed by Delayed Presentation of Mutilating Hand Injuries

Samir M. Kumta, MS, MCh (Plastic Surgery)[a],*,
Rajendra Nehete, MS, MCh, DNB (Plastic Surgery)[b],
Leena Jain, MS, MCh (Plastic Surgery)[c]

KEYWORDS

- Mutilating hand injuries • Late presentation • Debridement • Component loss in the hand
- Restoration of hand function

KEY POINTS

- Debridement and elimination of infection are the keys to success, with a multipronged strategy of radical debridement, early soft tissue cover, and appropriate antibiotic therapy.
- A detailed assessment and charting of intact structures is essential for planning further treatment; individualized treatment is essential.
- Skin cover with flaps is preferable to grafts. For complex reconstructions composite free flaps may be used.
- Adequate splinting and rest, combined with dynamic physiotherapy are required at all stages.

Man being naturally destitute of corporeal weapons, as also of any distinctive art, has received a compensation, in the gift of that particular instrument the hand, secondly is the gift of reason; by the employment of which gifts he arms and protects his body in every mode, and adorns his mind with the knowledge of every art

—*Galen[1]*

INTRODUCTION

In many parts of the world, a large number of patients with mangled hands receive incomplete or improper primary treatment, and eventually reach a specialist when they are unable to use the hand. Even in such instances, it is important to aim to obtain a hand that can perform basic functions and allow the individual to lead an independent life. According to Pinal, an acceptable hand is one with 3 fingers with near normal length, near normal sensation, and a functioning thumb.[2] This should serve as a basic benchmark for the reconstructive surgeon. Timing of presentation of hand injuries greatly influences the final outcome of hand function. Proper initial assessment is important to plan the sequence of reconstruction.[3]

The following features are commonly present in delayed presentation of mutilated hand injuries: inadequate initial assessment and patient counseling, inadequate debridement leading to infection, inappropriate stabilization of skeletal injuries, missed injuries, inadvertent ligation of vessels/nerves, a failure to recognize impending compartment syndrome, and improper mobilization resulting in stiffness.

Late presentations, apart from leading to poor functional outcome, also have a serious

---

Disclosure Statement: No Disclosures.
[a] Lilavati Hospital and Research Centre, Bandra Reclamation, Bandra West, Mumbai 400051, India; [b] Vedant Hospital, Shreehari Kute Marg, Nashik 422002, India; [c] Fortis Raheja Hospital, Mahim, Mumbai 400016, India
* Corresponding author. 1 Vikas, Bhagoji Keer Marg, Mahim, Mumbai 400016, India.
E-mail address: samir.kumta@gmail.com

Hand Clin 32 (2016) 569–583
http://dx.doi.org/10.1016/j.hcl.2016.07.008
0749-0712/16/© 2016 Elsevier Inc. All rights reserved.

socioeconomic impact on the patient and the family; most of the time, the patient himself is the sole breadwinner for the family. Multiple surgeries and a long duration of rehabilitation mean loss of work hours and wages. A prolonged absence from work may cause loss of job itself. Lack of financial or family support is one of the reasons for patients not complying with a rehabilitation protocol.

Pathophysiology of Hand Injuries in Delayed Presentation

Various factors affect the course of events, modalities of treatment, progress, results of treatment, and prognosis in patients who present late at the appropriate facility.[4] The nature of injury causes certain anatomic disruptions that in turn lead to functional deficits. Inadequate fixation results in malunion and nonunion secondarily affecting other joints and movement. Patients present with chronic pain, stiffness, malpositioning, scissoring, and sometimes severe deformities (**Fig. 1**). The onset of infection and secondary problems lead to certain sequelae (**Table 1**).

EVALUATION OF THE INJURED HAND

Evaluation of the injured hand starts with of obtaining a proper history and knowing the hand dominance and nature of job performed by the individual. Although one follows the same sequence of examination as when hand

injuries present early, in delayed presentation the assessment of loss in various tissue components can only be made at the time of debridement. Basic investigations like wound swabs for culture and antibiotic sensitivity, radiographs are done for all patients. Soft tissue ultrasound imaging, complex imaging like computed tomography or MRI, and assessment of vascular status by Doppler ultrasonography and angiography are done if necessary.[5–8]

Management

Proper assessment of damage is the cornerstone for planning the reconstruction of a mutilated hand injury. In delayed presentation, the usual tests may not be possible because of edema and pain owing to raw areas and inadequately stabilized bony injuries. So, the stage of debridement becomes even more critical in the overall management of the mutilated hand. This has to be done by a senior surgeon who will also be involved in the execution of the various stages of treatment and in the overall management until rehabilitation.

Debridement and Infection Control

Debridement is the key step for the prevention of infection. Often in delayed presentation, if the wound is already infected, radical debridement still is the key to success. The aim is to achieve primary healing of the wound. Debridement is considered conventionally to be removal of

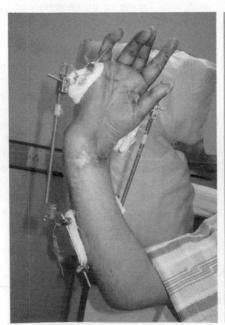
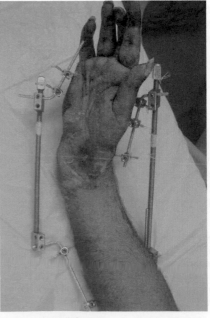

Fig. 1. Examples of malpositioning of bones owing to improper initial fixation of mangled hands.

Table 1
Sequelae seen in different tissues owing to delayed presentation of mutilated hand injuries

Structure	Altered Anatomy	Altered Physiology
Skin	Loss/retraction/ulcers/scars	Contractures
Skin grafts	Inadequate contracted graft, adherent to underlying structures	Primary and secondary contractures, restriction of movements
Scar	Immature, hypertrophic, inelastic, adherence to underlying structures, points of tenderness, direction	Excessive fibroblast proliferation, collagen deposition and fibrosis
Palmar fascia	Tightening/contraction	
Flexor tendon sheath	Contraction	
Flexor tendon	Shortening owing to loss Adhesions Loss of pulley system	Gliosis Quadriga effect Lumbrical plus finger Bowstringing
Extensor apparatus	Tendon adhesion Adhesion of dorsal capsule	Restriction of flexion extension lag Boutonniere deformity
Intrinsics	Contracture	
Ligament	Shortening of volar plate, collateral ligament and accessory collateral ligament	Joint contractures
Muscles	Devascularization or lack of nerve supply	Fibrosis Atrophy
Fascia	Interosseous membrane contracture in forearm causes restriction of pronation	
Web space	Contracture especially of first web	
Bone and joints	Malunion Nonunion with or without gap Arthritis–articular surface incongruity	
Nerve	Neuroma/muscle denervation	
Nails	Hook nail deformity/split nail/nonadherent nail	

necrotic tissue. In the current scenario, the hand surgeon must aim to leave behind only well-vascularized, viable tissue. That would involve excision of noncritical hypovascular structures in addition to removal of the obviously necrotic tissues. Debridement is carried out under tourniquet control to enable the surgeon to identify all structures and assess them individually.

In the hand, owing to the presence of several different tissues, it is important to sequentially debride each structure and assess the viability of residual tissues. Red dermis is unhealthy dermis and is trimmed until it is fresh yellow in color. Degloved skin flaps are trimmed to the line of viability. Muscle needs to be debrided sufficiently to prevent dead muscle from being a seat of infection. Contractility of muscle fibers is a good indicator of their viability. Tendon sheaths are checked for signs of tenosynovitis and drained optimally. Compartments need to be opened up to assess the viability of muscles and to prevent further damage owing to impending compartment syndrome secondary to inflammation or infection. Nerve and tendon ends are identified and tagged. Loose bone fragments and sequestra are removed. Conservation of bone fragments without any soft tissue attachment leads to infection and nonunion. If infection has caused loosening of implants used for bony fixation, the implants may have to be removed and alternative modes of fixation used. In these situations, we have found external fixators to be very useful.[9] One can consider replacement of implants only after infection control and an adequate soft tissue cover has been provided (**Fig. 2**).

In delayed presentation, a recheck after initial debridement is indicated within 48 hours to reassess viability of residual structures. Sequential debridement is the key in highly infected, contaminated, or doubtful cases. Serial debridements are carried out until all the necrotic tissues are cleared.

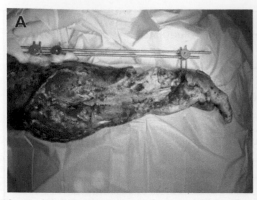
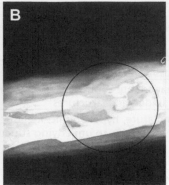
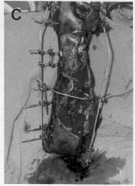

Fig. 2. (*A*) A badly infected forearm. (*B*) Antibiotic impregnated cement beads. (*C*) External stabilization and repeated thorough debridements eliminated the infection.

Once the bed seems to be healthy and local signs of inflammation subside, one may proceed for soft tissue cover. Negative pressure wound therapy is an adjunct to debridement for control of infection but never a substitute. It helps in the reduction of edema, improvement of vascularity, and reduction of inflammation. Long-duration intravenous antibiotics, repeated debridements, and local antibiotic therapy in the form of antibiotic-impregnated foam or bone cement are some of the strategies that may be necessary.

Management of Soft Tissue Cover

Patients who present late have lost a great deal of time and the ideal time for reconstruction has already passed. It is important to try and achieve maximum benefit through the minimum number of surgeries; thus, the timing of surgery now needs to be as early as possible. If the wound bed is good, bone and tendon reconstruction could be combined. Conventional strategy was to perform them in 3 stages—soft tissue coverage, bone reconstruction, and musculotendinous and nerve reconstruction. However, the present trend is to favor composite reconstruction (**Table 2**).

Adequate, pliable skin cover needs to be provided before reconstruction of all underlying tissues and this needs to be done as early as possible to hasten the subsequent steps in management and regress the duration of the pathophysiologic changes of the underlying tissues that would continue to occur. Replacement of grafts and scars with supple skin takes precedence above all reconstructions, primarily to provide a good soft tissue cover before replacement of tendons, bones, and joints so that these functionally important structures are well-covered. Good soft tissue cover reduces adhesions of reconstructed structures to allow their full range of movement. Excision of dense adherent scars,

release of contractures, and resurfacing with a pliable skin flap, either local regional or free, can be performed at the same time.

The selection of a pedicled or free flap is determined by the area to be covered and the availability of residual vessels in the hand and donor sites. Flaps of choice also vary depending on whether the volar or dorsal surface needs to be covered.

Table 2 Composite reconstruction of hand defects	
Osteocutaneous reconstruction	Free fibula with skin flap Lateral arm flap with humerus Scapular/parascapular free flap with scapula bone
Tenocutaneous reconstruction	Dorsalis pedis with vascularized tendon grafts Anterolateral thigh flap with fascia lata
Finger tips	Free toe pulp/hemipulp neurovascular island flaps
Nail bed	Free vascularized nail bed grafts
Glabrous skin flaps	Medial plantar artery free flap, medial plantar artery perforator free flap, free great/second toe pulp flap, toe hemi pulp flaps
Spare part surgery	Bone/tendon/nerve/skin grafts Free glabrous skin flaps Free nail bed grafts Free venous flow through flaps

For tissue resurfacing of small defects, numerous locoregional flaps have been described. Their use is minimal in mutilating injuries. For most major upper limb injuries, free flaps allowing resurfacing of large areas of the forearm and hand are the procedure of choice. Where multiple flaps are likely to be required, our approach is to reserve the microvascular reconstruction for the most important step, and do a pedicled flap for primary cover. For example, if skin resurfacing and a toe transfer are necessary, we prefer to do a pedicled groin, or an abdominal flap, and reserve the vessels for the more important toe transfer. Again, using free flaps have advantages of reducing the number of surgical steps especially when composite reconstructions are planned. If further procedures will be required beneath the flaps, skin flaps are our choice because they provide better access for secondary reconstruction.

We favor the superficial circumflex iliac artery flap for small to medium defects owing to its thin, pliable nature with negligible donor site morbidity. For a larger defect, we prefer a thin thoracodorsal artery perforator flap or suprafascial anterolateral thigh flap. Large suprafascial anterolateral thigh flaps, as large as 40 to 45 cm, have been described to survive well on a single perforator. For circumferential forearm and hand injuries, chimeric flaps may be needed like combined latissimus dorsi myocutaneous flap and serratus anterior flap, chimeric latissimus dorsi muscle flap and thoracodorsal artery perforator flap, or a combined anterolateral and anteromedial thigh flap. We have used a split latissimus dorsi on a few occasions to simultaneously cover isolated dorsal and volar defects on the hand or forearm (**Fig. 3**).

While resurfacing the dorsum of hand, aesthetics is an important consideration in flap selection owing to the unique nature of dorsal hand skin color, contour, and pliability. Venous flaps elevated in suprafascial flap are thin and pliable, and have been shown to give the best aesthetic outcome for small to medium sized defects in terms of color, contour, and texture match, requiring no debulking with minimal donor site morbidity without any sacrifice of a major artery. Venous flaps are usually taken from the forearm and size depends on venous anatomy of forearm.[10]

Fascial flaps from temporal, dorsal thoracic fascia, or anterolateral thigh fascia are remarkable for their pliability and provide an excellent color and contour match with split skin grafting for large dorsal defects done in a single stage along with minimal donor site morbidity.[11] However, fascial flaps often have the problem of graft loss, leading to unacceptable scarring.

Fasciocutaneous flaps like lateral arm flap or radial forearm flap are good for small to medium sized defects, but still require a secondary debulking and have an unsatisfactory donor site morbidity.[12] Partial muscle flaps like partial superior latissimus dorsi flap and medial rectus femoris flap involve only part of the muscle leaving behind a significant portion of the donor muscle with its nerve supply intact. These flaps are thin, do not require secondary thinning, and are indicated when there is a dead space, infection, or exposed hardware.[13,14]

Glabrous skin replacement for contact surfaces of hand where sensation is of primary importance, like the thumb or palm, can be done with medial plantar artery perforator flap causing no donor site morbidity while providing an excellent tissue match. The perforators are found running between the tendons of abductor hallucis and flexor hallucis brevis tendons and are followed to the medial plantar artery providing pedicle length of 3 to 4 cm.[15] The same benefits can also be obtained from free hemipulp toe flaps, but would suffice for relatively smaller areas of resurfacing. Toe pulp flaps can be harvested in a short time because only a small pedicle length is required and restore a satisfactory sensory recovery of 4 to 8 mm.[16]

Management of Bone

Bone problems associated with delayed presentations may be owing to infection of fractures, malunions, and nonunions. These can be avoided by adequate debridement and stable skeletal fixation. Small, loose bony fragments with questionable vascularity are often preserved by the primary treating surgeons with the hope that they will somehow survive and contribute to fracture union. However, these fragments are more often the source of infection and osteomyelitis. Debridement of infected bone is an often neglected necessity. Bone needs to be debrided to viable ends and the fracture stabilized suitably. In the upper limb, bone shortening and later distraction leads to imbalance between different muscle tendon units, stiffness, and loss of range of movement. Hence, if bone has to be removed it may be necessary to leave a gap and treat with vascularized bone grafts later. Untreated or improperly treated fractures need to be addressed earlier, before other tissues like nerves and tendons are reconstructed.

Small bone gaps can be treated with nonvascularized bone grafts, provided there is no active infection and there is a good soft tissue cover. Iliac crest, the fibula, distal radius, and olecranon are common bone graft donor sites. It is pertinent to

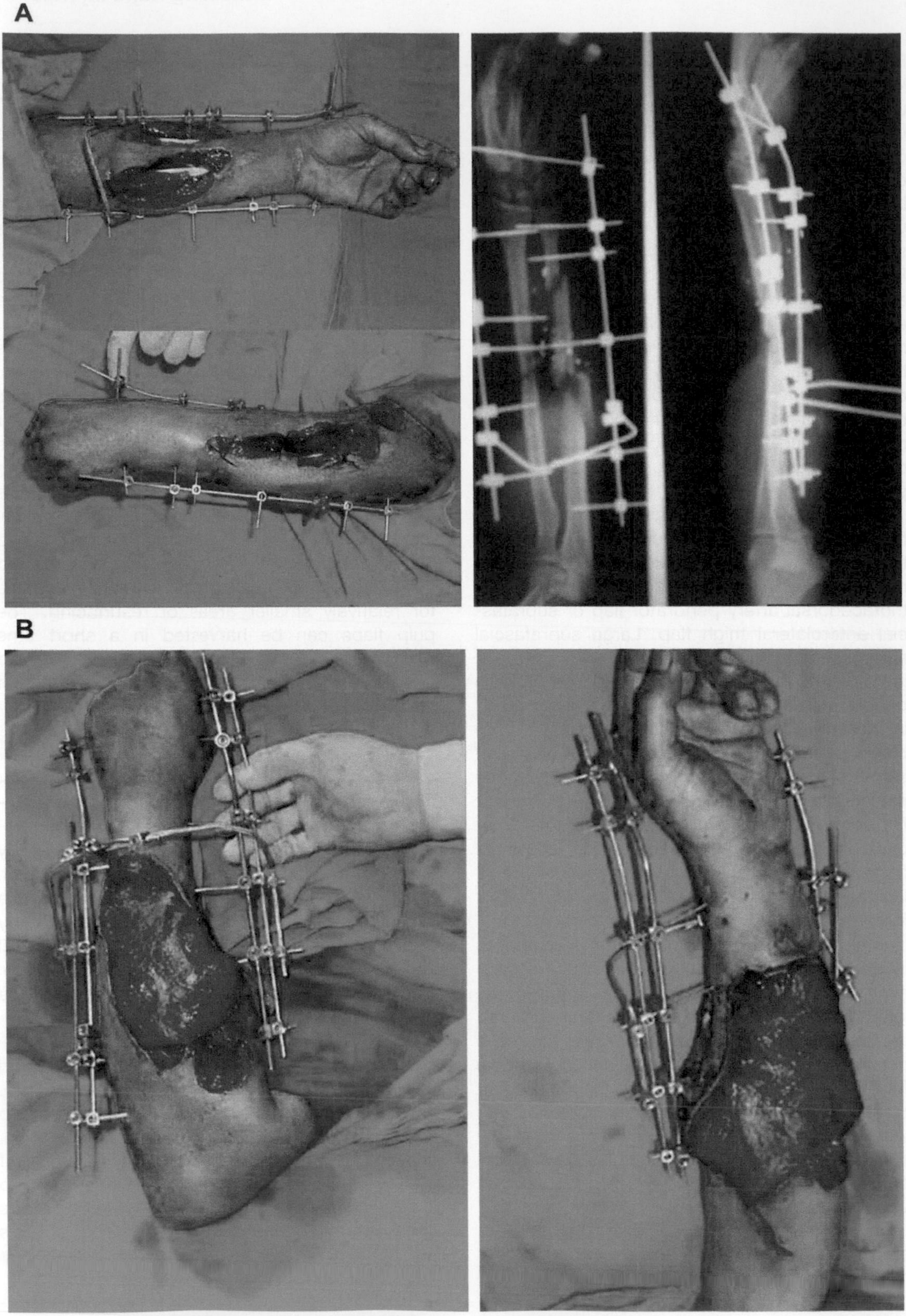

Fig. 3. An infected penetrating gunshot injury of the forearm with fractures of the radius and ulna and skin and soft tissue defects on both volar and dorsal aspects (*A*) was treated successfully by external stabilization, debridement, and then a split latissimus dorsi muscle flap (*B*). Subsequent bone grafting and tendon transfers for finger, thumb, and wrist extensors ensured excellent function (*C*).

C

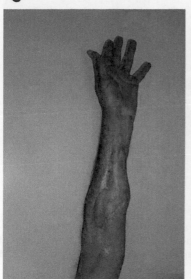 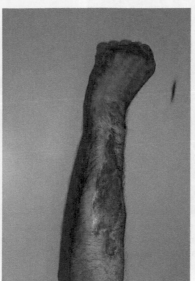 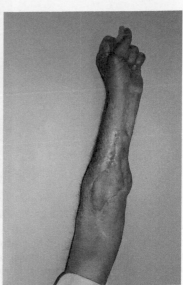

Fig. 3. (continued)

remember that nonvascularized bone grafts are associated with slow substitution, graft resorption, and failure to heal. Vascularized bone grafts allow cellular elements to survive with minimal graft necrosis and instant healing as well as remodeling.[17] Depending on the length of bone gaps, the choices for vascularized bone grafts are medial femoral condyle versus free fibular bone graft.

The medial femoral condyle vascularized bone graft has recently emerged as a useful corticoperiosteal bone graft for treatment of small gap nonunions in the upper limb, providing a small, thin, pliable, highly vascular tissue of optimal oseteogenic potential to conform into nonunions restoring them to timely union and improved function.[18] The medial femoral condyle is a rich donor site of 2 types of vascularized bone grafts with ease of harvest: corticoperiosteal vascularized small grafts based on highly vascular periosteal leash supplied by longitudinal branch of the descending genicular artery and osteoarticular/osteochondral vascularized graft based on transverse branch of osteoarticular branch of the descending genicular artery.[19] The former is used for phalanges and metacarpals where it can be wrapped around the nonunion and pegged between the bone ends of carpal nonunions; the latter is used for articular surface resurfacing of interphalangeal joints and metacarpophalangeal joints. Its use for radius and ulna nonunions has also been well-documented.[20] In the metacarpal area, iliac crest block grafts can be used to simultaneously

replace 2 or more metacarpals. Sometimes, innovative procedures like transverse peg grafts between adjacent proximal phalanges have been used to piggyback 1 finger with a missing joint onto the adjacent finger with a functioning joint, so as to allow both fingers to be moved simultaneously. Bony fixations are done using stainless steel wires, cannulated screws, or compression plates. For longer gaps, various composite flaps like serratus anterior muscle rib osteomycutaneous flap, iliac osteocutaneous flap, osteocutaneous scapula flap, dorsalis pedis osteocutaneous flap, and radial osteocutaneous free flap have been described for hand reconstruction; however, the free fibula flap has distinct advantages (**Fig. 4**). The double barrel fibula is useful for bridging bone gaps in the radius and ulna (**Fig. 5**). Providing 26 to 30 cm of cortical bone, to match metacarpal skeletal size, can be harvested safely without compromising the joints. The peroneal vessels run along the entire length of the fibula facilitating segmental osteotomies for reconstruction of adjacent or alternating metacarpal defects.[21] Its skin paddle is shown to be reliable even on a single perforator. Beside being thin and pliable, it matches the dorsal hand for composite reconstruction. The fibular flap provides a better option for 1-stage composite tissue and simultaneous functional tendon reconstruction.[22] Another potential use of the fibula in composite reconstructions is its use as a flow through flap for anastomosis of vessels of a simultaneous toe transfer or muscle transfer.[23]

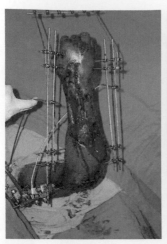
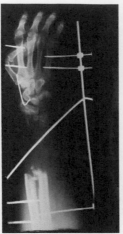
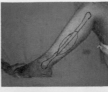
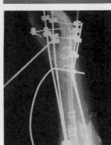
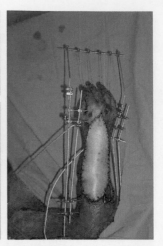

Fig. 4. A 35-year-old driver lost the distal half of his radius and ulna after a road traffic accident. After failed attempts to heal the wound by grafting, he was referred to us. After thorough initial debridement and change of external fixation, a fibula osteocutaneous flap was done to bridge the gap in the forearm bones and convert it into a single bone forearm. The bone united successfully.

Joint defects can be reconstructed with autogenous osteochondral grafts to avoid arthrodesis and can be taken from the second, third, or fourth metatarsophalangeal joint, even from the injured hand itself. Pedicled osteoarticular flaps can be harvested from the hamate or capitate to reconstruct defects of the intraarticular part of the proximal phalanx, or a third metacarpal base osteoarticular flap for the reconstruction of metacarpophalangeal joint defects.

Management of Nerves

Neuroma excision and neurolysis can be done simultaneously with other procedures because no mobilization is required. Nerve gaps can be grafted at this time as well. Chronically injured nerves become stiffer with about 50% reduction in elasticity, implying the need for nerve grafts for delayed repairs. Fibrosis of the nerve ends prevents approximation of the severed nerve ends; hence, nerve grafting is required even though there is no loss of nerve tissue because 15% elongation of nerve causes complete ischemia. The recovery of sensation is aimed at preventing cutaneous ulcers and restoring by at least restoring protective sensation.[24] Being surrounded by gliding tissue, normal nerves have enough longitudinal excursions with limb flexion and extension, whereas a nerve graft becomes adherent to the recipient bed during vascularization; thus, when subjected to longitudinal stretch, the nerve and repair come under tension. The harvested graft must be long enough to span the nerve gap without tension while the adjacent joints are extended. This should also be the position of temporary postoperative immobilization.

Priority areas for restoration of sensations are to the ulnar side of the thumb, the radial side of the index finger, and the ulnar border of the hand.

Management of the Musculotendinous Unit

For optimal management of the musculotendinous unit, prerequisites include a stable soft tissue cover, supple scars, stable skeleton, and supple joints. Metacarpophalangeal joint capsulotomies are often required at this stage. Joint contractures are caused by decreased motion, splinting position, volar plate scarring, bowstringing, adhesions, skin contracture, and ligament contracture. Early recognition and continued follow-up with a hand therapist for splint adjustment are crucial to prevent the establishment of contracture. Release should proceed systematically, sequentially releasing contracted structures until full extension is reached. This again needs to be followed by intensive physiotherapy until all joints are supple; this is a fundamental prerequisite to tendon tenolysis, tendon grafts, or transfers.[25]

The timing of tendon reconstruction or transfer is generally about 3 months after the soft tissue cover, once the scars become supple. During this waiting period, passive physiotherapy of joints is essential. Tendon trauma (from initial injury and intraoperative handling), an irregular bunched up repair, and postoperative immobilization all facilitate the formation of adhesions. Thus, tenolysis is indicated when passive range of motion is nearly normal or greater than active range of motion, with supple tissues and healed fractures. It should be performed carefully with sharp dissection, as established scarring makes tenolysis difficult and may cause a tendon to rerupture. Tendon and

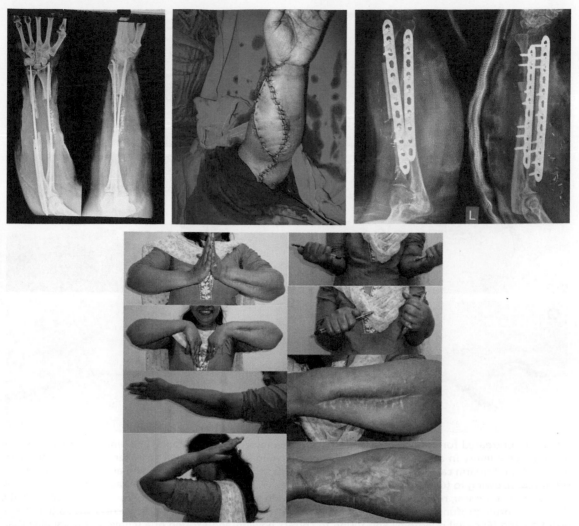

Fig. 5. A 40-year-old lady with gap nonunion of radius and ulna was successfully treated with a fibular osteocutaneous flap. Despite loss of part of the fibular skin island, the bones united within 6 months.

pulleys may be densely scarred and/or swollen. In such cases, tenolysis may not be helpful. A secondary flexor tendon reconstruction with grafts is a better option.[26] Tendon reconstruction is done using tendon grafts with tension adjustment to keep the joints in functional position. Grafts include unilateral or bilateral palmaris longus tendon, plantaris tendon, fascia lata, and extensor slips. For long gaps, multiple donor sites are used for tendon grafts. Reconstruction with grafts can be done in a single stage or in stages with prior creation of synovial pseudosheath using silicon rods, depending on the extent of scarring of underlying bed. When tendon repair is attempted several months after injury, tendon ends are distorted, tendon sheath is fibrosed, muscle tendon unit is shortened owing to myostatic contracture, and proximal cut muscle is often found to have retracted and atrophied so much that it has lost it's elasticity and contractility and adheres to the surrounding tissue. In such situations, bridging the gap with tendon grafts often does not produce the desired range of movement. Tendon transfers work better in these situations (**Fig. 6**). Hence, a detailed charting of donor nerves and muscle tendon units is essential to determine available motors for tendon transfers without causing significant functional deficits. Tenolysis or tendon transfers must be followed by suitable physiotherapy.

Tendon transfers require a good soft tissue cover, full passive range of motion of all joints, expendable donors of power more than 4, straight line of pull and synergistic function. Merits of tendon transfer include return of function soon after the immobilization period (within 4–6 weeks).

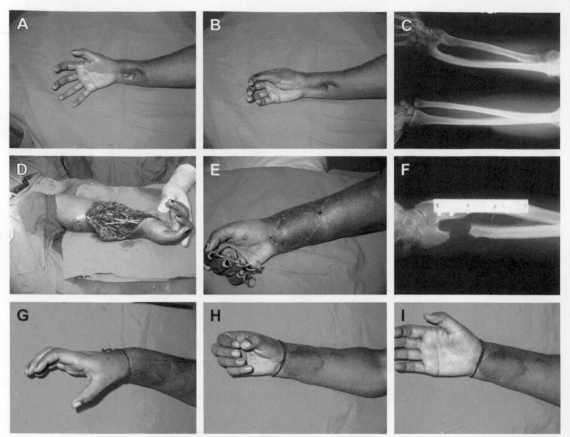

Fig. 6. An untreated forearm injury with fractures of the lower end of the radius and ulna, flexor tendons, and median nerve injury in a 20 year-old-woman. (*A*) The wound had healed with an adherent scar over the volar aspect of the forearm causing loss of finger flexion, (*B*) bowing of the ulna and radius, and inability to supinate the forearm, owing to (*C*) radioulnar synostosis at the lower end, with malunion of the radius and ulna fractures. (*D*) Excision of the scar, release of all adhesions, and tendon transfer from the extensor carpi radialis longus to the flexor digitorum profundus tendons, median nerve grafting followed by (*E*) soft tissue cover with a thin lateral arm flap and (*F*) radial osteotomy and fusion to correct bowing, and excision of a segment of distal ulna (Darrach's procedure) to allow supination. (*G*) With this 1-stage composite reconstruction, the dense scar was replaced with pliable and aesthetic skin cover. (*H*) Finger flexion was restored, hand sensations and thumb function were restored and (*I*) supination was restored.

However, some of the disadvantages include extensive dissection, postoperative immobilization, adhesion formation, and potential inadequacy of the tendon–muscle balance. In a systematic review of the literature, early active motion protocols seemed to have the best intersection of low rupture rates and improved range of motion with tendon repair, reconstruction and transfers.[27]

In composite injuries of tendon and nerve, one can choose between nerve or tendon transfer depending on the time of presentation. There are time-dependent, irreversible changes that occur in the motor end plates; thus, the longer the duration of denervation, the lesser the chances of reinnervation. The optimal time of surgical intervention with nerve transfers depends on the distance of the repair from the target muscle. The time taken

by the regenerating nerve to reach the target muscles should be well within the usual survival of the denervated motor endplates, which is approximately 18 months. Any regenerating nerve arriving at a motor end plate after this period may not be functionally useful. Loss of time will only leave us with the option of tendon transfer or a microvascular transfer of a functioning muscle.

The goal of nerve transfers is to restore function by transferring a functional but less important nerve to a distal but more important denervated nerve, thereby minimizing the time to reinnervation. Certain prerequisites before nerve transfer include appropriate donor nerve in the vicinity of the motor endplate of the target muscle, with a large number of motor axons to donate while still supplying the native muscle, a good size match to the recipient nerve, and synergistic function to the motor function of the muscle to be reconstructed. Nerve transfers have reliable outcomes and fewer cocontraction issues; dissection is in unscarred tissue planes while avoiding disruption of the tendon–muscle unit balance. Incomplete recovery and difficult motor retraining are its demerits.[28]

In low median neuropathy, the terminal branch of anterior interosseous nerve is transferred to the median recurrent motor branch with an interpositional nerve graft. For high median neuropathies, transfers include radial nerve branches to the supinator and extensor carpi radialis brevis transferred into the anterior interosseous nerve and pronator teres branches of the median nerve or nerve branch to brachialis can be transferred into anterior interosseous nerve. For the ulnar nerve, the terminal branch of the anterior interosseous nerve is transferred to the deep ulnar motor nerve branch. Nerve transfers advocated for radial nerve are nerve branches of flexor digitorum superficialis to the extensor carpi radialis brevis, nerve branches of the flexor carpi radialis and palmaris longus to the posterior interosseous nerve or ulnar nerve–innervated branch of the flexor carpi ulnaris to the posterior interosseous nerve.

If there are no available motors as donors or if there is loss of proximal muscles, functioning muscle transfers may be performed. Functioning muscles for hand are free muscle transfers like gracilis or serratus anterior muscle flap.

In mangled injuries, the standard transfers are often not possible and one needs to individualize depending on what is available after a detailed muscle and nerve charting. Further, in cases of combined nerve injuries, the available donor muscles are limited and one needs to prioritize functions to be preserved and restored before embarking on nerve and tendon transfers. This is best done by considering the patient's desires and needs (**Fig. 7**).

Reconstruction of Thumb and Digits

In late reconstructions with loss of digits, the primary debridement has an important bearing on the functional and aesthetic outcome of transferred toes. Preservation of as much possible healthy viable lengths of bone, tendon, vessels, and nerves helps in avoiding the need for tendon and vessel grafts.[29] Presence of skin cover and a wide first web are prerequisites to thumb and digit reconstruction.

For thumb reconstruction, one can choose between great toe transfer and lesser toe transfer; however, great toe transfer and its variants give better results.[30] The variants include wraparound toe transfer or trimmed toe transfer for reconstruction of thumb amputations distal to the metacarpal neck.[31] Proximal to metacarpal neck in the presence of active thenar muscles, interposition bone graft with toe transfer, or transmetatarsal second toe transfer would be required. In the absence of thenar muscles, a secondary opponensplasty can be performed after toe transfer. In cases of a damaged carpometacarpal joint, an immobile thumb post is created with a great toe or second toe transfer. Single digit reconstruction with toe transfers is a disputed procedure, especially in the nondominant hand. Depending on the level of digital amputation, options available are toe pulp transfers, partial lesser toe transfers, wrap-around toe transfers, and total lesser toe transfers. In the management of multiple digit amputations, reconstruction of at least 2 adjacent digits is important to provide a useful tripod pinch, lateral stability, a hook grip, and precision.[32]

The radial 2 digits are important for fine manipulation and thus global hand function, and the ulnar 2 digits are important for a powerful grasp. In general, a hand with 2 long fingers and a thumb of normal length is considered as functionally superior to a hand with 3 long fingers and a shortened thumb, especially in terms of fine motor or precision handling ability.[33]

Reconstruction of a metacarpal hand is determined by the level of digital amputation. Distal to the web space, amputations can be reconstructed with bilateral second toe transfers and amputations proximal to that are reconstructed with combined second and third toe transfers.[34] With an intact metacarpal articular surface, combined second and third toes would be transferred, whereas a damaged articular surface would require a transmetatarsal-level transfer of toes.[35]

The ultimate goal in hand reconstruction is not just to preserve nonselectively all living tissue, but rather to restore function.[36] Pollicization of a nonfunctional index finger restores sensate, functional, opposable thumb, and a widened first web space. This reduces time to rehabilitation and, more important, eliminates nonfunctional tissues that may interfere with normal coordinated movements. In multidigital injuries, other injured fingers can also be pollicized. Ray transfers use optimal reconstruction of a reduced number of remaining fingers, and as do ray amputations with metacarpal transfer.[37]

Tertiary surgeries

After skin resurfacing, bony stability, and motorization are achieved, patients are reassessed for the level of function achieved. At this stage, restrictive pathology often needs to be treated.

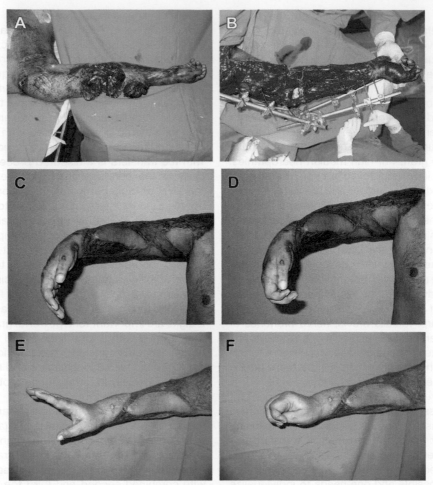

Fig. 7. (*A*) An extensive crush injury with skin degloving, severe muscle damage, fractures around the elbow, and rupture of brachial vessels in a 40-year-old man involved in a road traffic accident. (*B*) Thorough debridement and external stabilization of the fractures with repair of the brachial vessels. (*C*) Skin cover was obtained with a pedicled latissimus dorsi flap and skin grafts to cover the entire area. Complete healing of all wounds was achieved in 6 weeks. (*D*) After all wounds had healed, the patient was unable to extend his fingers and thumb, and had an ankylosed elbow. (*E, F*) After assessment of available muscles for transfer, the flexor carpi ulnaris was transferred to the extensor digitorum and the flexor superficialis of the middle finger was transferred to the extensor carpi radialis brevis to restore complete hand function. Arthrolysis of the elbow was also performed.

Restriction of forearm supination is a common problem that is treated by either a Sauve Kapandji or Darrach procedure. Fractures close to the joints or intraarticular fractures frequently result in painful or stiff joints. Arthrodesis of such joints may need to be performed when they are refractory to attempts at arthrolysis. Debulking of flaps and scar revisions are the last procedures performed after functional rehabilitation is complete.

Last, for patients whose hand is so badly damaged that no useful function is probable may be better served by amputation than by persistent attempts at salvage.[38] Numerous factors influence the decision to amputate, including the extent of tissue damage, pain, infection, appearance, functional requirements, economics, safety, and the psychological makeup of the patient. Whenever a decision to amputate is taken, or forced by circumstances, care must be taken to ensure that the best possible stump be provided for future prosthetic fitment, or possible limb transplantation. In these situations, free flaps have been found to be useful to preserve stump length (**Fig. 8**).

The patient must be informed of what is possible, probable, and feasible if salvage is to be pursued; both the patient and the surgeon must have a clear understanding of the practical and psychological aspects of amputation.

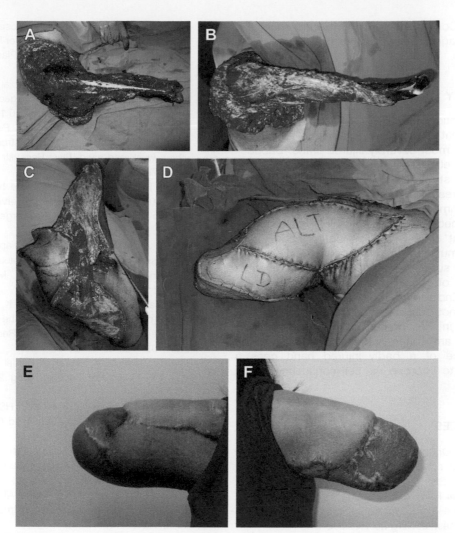

Fig. 8. When all is lost: when a limb is amputated, care needs to be taken to provide the best possible amputation stump. (*A, B*) This 14-year-old girl lost her upper limb in a road accident, and the residual upper arm stump was completely degloved. (*C, D*) After thorough debridement, the stump was covered with 2 flaps, a pedicled latissimus dorsi myocutaneous flap from the back, and a free anterolateral thigh flap to provide good robust skin cover to the humerus all around. (*E, F*) A well-covered stump allows the prosthetic limb to fit well.

Approximately 2 weeks after the amputation, the stump will be healed and ready for fitting with an intermediate prosthesis with an elastomer foam socket. This prosthesis allows a free elbow and functions the same as the definitive prosthesis, which has a rigid socket and can be fitted whenever the stump has healed and contracted.

Finally, because hand transplant programs have now evolved the world over with successful results, hand transplantation may eventually be considered for severely mutilated hands when a breakthrough in transplant immunology occurs.[39]

REHABILITATION

At initial presentation, patients usually have considerable joint stiffness and restricted range of movement. Until the soft tissue contracture is released, physiotherapy does not offer much benefit. However, after release of scar and contractures, and resurfacing with a pliable flap, the situation often changes dramatically. At this stage, a vigorous rehabilitation program helps to restore passive movements. At this stage, tendon grafts or transfers may be performed, and then the rehabilitation process is recommenced. Intelligent use of simple splints aid in the mobilization process. Compression garments and scar care with massage are essential for at least 6 months to 1 year.

SUMMARY

A systematic treatment plan individualized for each patient can restore reasonable function in all but the most severely injured limbs. Debridement and elimination of infection are the most important steps in commencing treatment in delayed presentation of mutilating injuries of the hand. Alignment and stabilization of bones should be performed as early as possible. There is an old adage that says that flaps are preferred over grafts in mutilating injuries, because they allow secondary surgery on underlying structures, protect repair of critical structures, and prevent adhesions. End-to-end repair of injured structures is usually not possible in delayed presentation of mutilating injuries presenting late, and grafts or transfers are often required. Restoring the appearance of a badly injured hand goes a long way to improve the self-confidence of the patient.

REFERENCES

1. Kidd J. On the adaptation of external nature to the physical condition of man. London: H. G. Bohn; 1852. p. 28.
2. del Piñal F. Severe mutilating injuries to the hand: Guidelines for organizing the chaos. J Plast Reconstr Aesthet Surg 2007;60:816–27.
3. Alphonsus CK. Principles in the management of a mangled hand. Indian J Plast Surg 2011;44:219–26.
4. Jones LA. The assessment of hand function: a critical review of techniques. J Hand Surg Am 1989; 14:221–8.
5. Lister GD. Local flaps to the hand. Hand Clin 1985;1: 621–40.
6. Ghori AK, Chung KC. The medical Doppler in hand surgery: its scientific basis, applications, and the history of its namesake, Christian Johann Doppler. J Hand Surg Am 2007;32(10):1595–9.
7. Klein MB, Karanas YL, Chow LC, et al. Early experience with computed tomographic angiography in microsurgical reconstruction. Plast Reconstr Surg 2003;112:498–503.
8. Koman LA, Ruch DS, Smith BP, et al. Vascular disorders. In: Green DP, Hotchkiss RN, Pederson WC, et al, editors. Green's operative hand surgery. Philadelphia: Elsevier; 2005. p. 2265–313.
9. Freeland AE, Jabaley ME. Stabilization of fractures in the hand and wrist with traumatic soft tissue and bone loss. Hand Clin 1988;4(3):425–36.
10. Woo SH, Kim KC, Lee GJ, et al. A retrospective analysis of 154 arterialized venous flaps for hand reconstruction: An 11-year experience. Plast Reconstr Surg 2007;119:1823–38.
11. Carty MJ, Taghinia A, Upton J. Fascial flap reconstruction of the hand: a single surgeon's 30-year experience. Plast Reconstr Surg 2010;125:953–62.
12. Jones NF, Jarrahy R, Kaufman MR. Pedicled and free radial forearm flaps for reconstruction of the elbow, wrist, and hand. Plast Reconstr Surg 2008; 121:887–98.
13. Brooks D, Buntic RF. Partial muscle harvest: Our first 100 cases attempting to preserve form and function at the donor site. Microsurgery 2008;28: 606–11.
14. Chang J, Jones N. Muscle free flaps with full-thickness skin grafting: Improved contour over traditional musculocutaneous free flaps. Microsurgery 2001;21:70–3.
15. Koshima I, Urushibara K, Inagawa K, et al. Free medial plantar perforator flaps for the resurfacing of finger and foot defects. Plast Reconstr Surg 2001;107:1753–8.
16. Lee DC, Kim JS, Ki SH, et al. Partial second toe pulp free flap. Plast Reconstr Surg 2008;121(3): 898–907.
17. Khan SN, Cammisa FP Jr, Sandhu HS, et al. The biology of bone grafting. J Am Acad Orthop Surg 2005;13(1):77–86.
18. Doi K, Sakai K. Vascularised periosteal bone graft from the supracondylar region of the femur. Microsurgery 1994;5:305–15.
19. Friedrich J, Pederson WC, Bishop AT, et al. New workhorse flaps in hand reconstruction. Hand 2012;7:45–54.
20. Jones DB, Moran SL, Bishop AT, et al. Free-vascularized medial femoral condyle bone transfer in the treatment of scaphoid nonunions. Plast Reconstr Surg 2010;125:1176–84.
21. Yajima H, Tamai S, Ono H, et al. Free vascularised fibula grafts in surgery of the upper limb. J Reconstr Microsurg 1999;15:515.
22. Lin CH, Wei FC, Chen HC, et al. Outcome comparison in traumatic lower-extremity reconstruction by using various composite vascularised bone transplantation. Plast Reconstr Surg 1999; 104:984.
23. Lee HB, Tark KC, Kang SY, et al. Reconstruction of composite metacarpal defects using a fibula free flap. Plast Reconstr Surg 2000;105:1448.
24. Slutsky DJ. The management of digital nerve injuries. J Hand Surg Am 2014;39:1208–15.
25. Momeni A, Grauel E, Chang J. Complications after flexor tendon injuries. Hand Clin 2010;26: 179–89.
26. Tang JB. Indications, methods, postoperative motion and outcome evaluation of primary flexor

tendon repairs in Zone 2. J Hand Surg Eur Vol 2007; 32:118–29.

27. Chesney A, Chauhan A, Kattan A, et al. Systematic review of flexor tendon rehabilitation protocols in zone II of the hand. Plast Reconstr Surg 2011;127: 1583–92.

28. Mackinnon SE, Humphreys DB. Nerve transfers. Oper Tech Plast Reconstr Surg 2002;9:89–99.

29. Wei FC. Tissue preservation in hand injury: the first step in toe to hand transplantation. Plast Reconstr Surg 1998;102:2497–501.

30. Muzaffar AR, Chao JJ, Friedrich JB. Posttraumatic thumb reconstruction. Plast Reconstr Surg 2005; 116:103e–22e.

31. Morrison WA, O'Brien BM, MacLeod AM. Thumb reconstruction with a free neurovascular wrap-around flap from the big toe. J Hand Surg Am 1980;5:575–83.

32. Wei FC, Colony LH, Chen HC, et al. Combined second and third toe transfer. Plast Reconstr Surg 1989; 84:651–61.

33. Wei FC, Chen HC, Chuang CC, et al. Microsurgical thumb reconstruction with toe transfer: selection of various techniques. Plast Reconstr Surg 1994;93: 345–51 [discussion: 352–7].

34. Tsai TM, McCabe S, Beatty ME. Second toe transfer for thumb reconstruction in multiple digit amputations including thumb and basal joint. Microsurgery 1987;8:146–53.

35. Wilhelmi BJ, Lee WP, Pagenstert GI, et al. Replantation in the mutilated hand. Hand Clin 2003;19:89–120.

36. Bravo CJ, Horton T, Moran SL, et al. Traumatized index finger pollicization for thumb reconstruction. J Hand Surg Am 2008;33:257–62.

37. Neuhaus V, Nagy L, Jupiter JB. Bone loss in the hand. J Hand Surg 2013;38A:1032–9.

38. Brown PW. Sacrifice of the unsatisfactory hand. J Hand Surg 1979;4(5):417–23.

39. Amirlak B, Gonzalez R, Gorantla V, et al. Creating a hand transplant program. Clin Plast Surg 2007; 34(2):279–89.

Pushing the Boundaries of Salvage in Mutilating Upper Limb Injuries
Techniques in Difficult Situations

S. Raja Sabapathy, MS (Gen), MCh (Plastic), DNB (Plastic), FRCS (Edin), MAMS[a],*,
David Elliot, MA, BM BCh, FRCS[b],
Hari Venkatramani, MS, MCh (Plastic), DNB (Plastic), EDHS (Euro. Board)[a]

KEYWORDS

- Bilateral upper limb amputation • Free functioning muscle transfer • Flow through free flap
- Toe transfers • Mutilating hand injuries

KEY POINTS

- Even in most severe injuries of the upper limb, with the current available reconstructive armamentarium basic function can almost always be restored.
- In multilevel digital amputations, heterotopic replantation and rearrangement of parts can result in useful function.
- Even in most severe combined injuries with tissue loss of the proximal upper limb, if the hand is structurally intact it is worth salvaging. Free functioning muscle transfer can restore useful function.
- The more the mutilation, the more the conservation of parts. Salvage of skeletal segments and joints may prove useful in subsequent reconstruction particularly in bilateral injuries.
- Multistaged reconstruction is almost the rule. Timing and sequence of the procedures are key to success.

INTRODUCTION

When a surgeon is faced with a mutilated upper limb, the goal of management is to aim to obtain as good a functioning upper limb as his or her surgical experience and imagination can envisage. At times, a variety of factors, including the severity of the injury, will thwart this goal and the bar must be lowered to obtain, at the very least, enough basic function to enable the individual to perform the basic activities of living and lead an independent life. In the authors' opinion, this can always be achieved by surgeons with experience in this field.

In the acute situation and, sometimes later, particularly if circumstances force a lowering of the bar, the question arises: salvage or amputate? Unlike with the lower limb under these circumstances, there are no validated and acceptable scoring systems to guide the surgeon dealing with complex upper limb injuries. At present, the bias should always be toward salvage because the alternative means rehabilitation with a prosthesis and upper limb prostheses remain far from ideal.[1–5] For the lower limb, prostheses have a simpler task and work well. Not so with our current upper limb prostheses.[6–8] However, more

Disclosure statement: The authors have nothing to disclose.
[a] Department of Plastic, Hand & Reconstructive Microsurgery and Burns, Ganga Hospital, 313, Mettupalayam Road, Coimbatore, Tamil Nadu 641 043, India; [b] Department of Plastic Surgery, St Andrews Centre for Plastic Surgery and Burns, Broomfield Hospital, Court Road Broomfield, Chelmsford, Essex CM1 7ET, UK
* Corresponding author.
E-mail address: rajahand@gmail.com

Hand Clin 32 (2016) 585–597
http://dx.doi.org/10.1016/j.hcl.2016.06.003
0749-0712/16/© 2016 Elsevier Inc. All rights reserved.

sophisticated upper limb prostheses are being developed and may change this balance in the future.[9] The third option of hand transplantation is evolving surgically but retains the same long-term immune problems, awaiting useful advances in this field.[10,11]

Three factors have a bearing on the ultimate outcome following major upper limb injury: (1) patient-related factors, (2) injury-related factors, and (3) surgeon-related factors. The patient factors of age-associated comorbidities, coincidental injuries, work status, family support, social security status, and personal motivation are as always. The complexity of the injury to the upper limb per se and the time from injury to reaching an appropriate surgical facility are the two injury-related factors that have the most bearing on the outcome. As surgeons, we have little control over these factors, with the exception of speeding progress from the first telephone call to the anesthetic anteroom of our operating theater, particularly through our own hospital. Ultimately, the factors that most influence the outcome are surgeon related, namely, the skills and experience of the surgical team, their attitude toward salvage, and the infrastructure of the service. A skilled surgical team in a supportive infrastructure can make a very big difference to the outcome.[12] Available techniques, and knowledge of these, are most important and attention to detail is crucial. Almost always, the treatment plan has to be individualized. However, experienced senior surgeons will draw on their direct experience of previous cases and the more universal discussion of such cases internationally, both in meetings and in the literature of the last 40 years.[13,14]

This article uses a few cases to illustrate the thinking the authors use in such cases and illustrates the development of appropriate plans of management. These cases remain individual cases but aim to guide the reader in how to plan when faced with complex primary and secondary upper limb injuries. The article deals with instances of bilateral amputations and extensive unilateral injuries involving combined tissue losses. They came to the authors following road traffic accidents and industrial disasters, such as power press injuries, explosive blasts, and electrical burns.

BASIC PRINCIPLES

1. When there is extensive loss due to amputation in the upper limb, every effort is made to conserve the available parts, both those attached and those freed by the injury from patients. The greater the mutilation, the more the urgency to conserve all that is living and all that is undamaged.[15] This conservation should include attempts to preserve all attached parts at the start of surgery and all amputated parts for as long as necessary to allow surgical salvage by either cooling or by revascularization, in an appropriate position or ectopically. Nothing with potential to be used, either whole or as component spare parts, should be discarded during debridement.[16–20]

2. Primary healing of the wound should be a goal. When the wound heals primarily, the stage is set for success. Radical debridement and early soft tissue cover achieve this.[21,22]

3. Strong skeletal, tendon, and, if possible, nerve reconnections must be made. When the skeleton is badly disorganized, any fixation with which the surgeon is comfortable can be used but must be sufficiently strong to allow relatively early mobilization.[23] The same is true of the tendon sutures, particularly of the flexors. Early mobilization is necessary to counter the enormous fibrin edema of such injuries and avoid the gluing effect of the fibrin-to-scar conversion, which follows all such injuries and can lead to a living limb, which is functionally little more than a paperweight.

4. The available structures should be placed or replaced in the optimum position of function to be useful later. This point is particularly the case with the first ray: utmost care must be taken to keep the thumb in the ideal position.[24,25] It must be stabilized in abduction and in line with the outer border of the index finger in a slightly pronated position irrespective of whether there is adequate soft tissue cover or not. Most cases of crush and blast injuries destroy the thenar muscles, so provision of soft tissue cover without the convenience of the thenar muscles is not uncommon. Unless the position of the thumb is maintained as earlier, the fibrosis that follows these injuries to the first web space leads to web contracture, which is very difficult to correct later. The authors prevent this by either using axial K wiring or by bending a K wire in the form of a V and placing it to hold the first web space open for several months after the injury (**Fig. 1**).[26] With the thumb in a good position, soft tissue cover is provided.[27] With the thumb held out in this optimum position, flap requirement is much greater than with the first web closed.[28] Compromise here will result in contracture of the first web. Important also, if there is proximal skeletal injury, is that the forearm is stabilized and plastered with the forearm in the supinated position. It is easier to apply pedicled flaps to the supinated forearm.[29] Rehabilitation is also

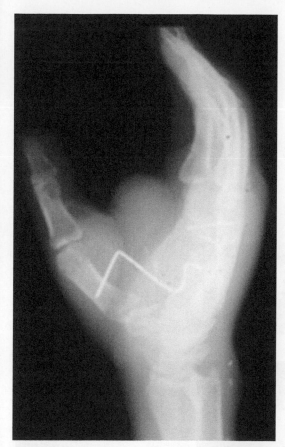

Fig. 1. Retaining the first web space by a bent K wire until wound healing is essential to obtain a good outcome. (*From* Lees VC, Wren C, Elliot D. Internal splints for prevention of first web contracture following severe disruption of the first web space. J Hand Surg Br 1994;19:561; with permission.)

easier in this forearm position and function is also greater. A forearm fixed in pronation is extremely difficult to rehabilitate and will have poor function.

5. Soft tissue cover with flaps is not only necessary to achieve primary healing. Flaps must cover joints bereft of soft tissue cover if the joint is to be retained functionally.[30] Flaps are used for immediate conduits in replantation and immediate toe transfer.[31,32] They also facilitate late finger reconstructions, including toe transfer.[33–36] Pedicled flaps, local and distant, allow closure of amputations at all levels but particularly at the bases of proximal phalanges in the metacarpal hand and at the wrist in transmetacarpal amputations, without further shortening.

Some of these technical considerations are illustrated in the complex reconstructions described later.

MULTILEVEL AMPUTATIONS IN THE HAND

A 16-year-old art student doing a summer holiday job injured his right hand in a power saw. The hand hit the saw twice, resulting in double-level cut injury to the ulnar 3 fingers and total amputation of the index finger and thumb (**Fig. 2**A). The amputated thumb was not salvageable. With all the fingers amputated, the hand needed reconstruction. Debridement is an important part of replantation.[37,38] Detailed examination of the amputated parts and proximal segment revealed that not all the parts could be used. Relatively uninjured segments were isolated and prepared for replantation (see **Fig. 2**B). The thumb was destroyed, and the authors used the ring finger as a thumb. To make a wider first web space, the index finger was replaced on the ring metacarpal and the middle finger on the little metacarpal and the tip of the discarded little finger was replanted on top of the middle to replace the missing tip and bring it out to length (see **Fig. 2**C). Trimming the bone stumps and using the available skin provided a good wide first web.[39] The boy functionally recovered well and went back to art school, graduated, and is now working as a commercial artist (see **Fig. 2**D).

Discussion

When a patient with multiple level amputations presents, one may be overwhelmed by the complexity of the reconstruction needed.[40] Instead of thinking of anatomic reconstruction, one needs to think of functional reconstruction. Use of available segments in heterotopic situations and salvage of tissues as spare parts are the key to success.[16,18] In the hand it starts with the reconstruction of the thumb.[31] Adequate length, stability, and sensation are the main parameters to be gained.[24,25] In the presented case, the distal part of the ring was used to reconstruct the thumb. In the thumb, the ulnar side digital artery is always bigger than the radial side, and, so, in a major injury it is preferentially isolated and repaired. Similarly, the authors have found that the vessels on the inner side of the border digits are bigger. So when replanting the index, the ulnar side digital artery and the radial side digital artery in the little finger are preferentially repaired. Success in replantation in major injuries so much depends on choosing a proximal vessel with good blood flow. If the blood vessels at the base of the thumb are not satisfactory, the authors do not hesitate to use a vein graft bridging the radial artery in the anatomic snuffbox and the ulnar side digital artery of the thumb.[16] Positioning the thumb for the distal anastomosis can be an issue. This issue can be overcome by making the distal anastomosis in

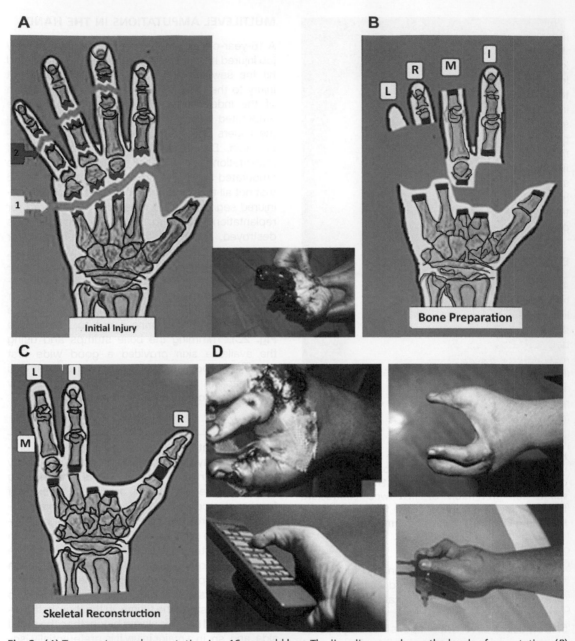

Fig. 2. (*A*) Transmetacarpal amputation in a 16-year-old boy. The line diagram shows the levels of amputation. (*B*) The picture shows segments that were found usable. (*C*) The pattern of reconstruction by rearrangement of parts. (*D*) Long-term result of reconstruction showing a usable hand. I, index; L, little; M, middle; R, ring.

the bench or by viewing the anastomosis site from the dorsum. Orienting the replanted thumb is critical for success. Because, in this situation, thenar muscles are available, good function can be achieved. The chosen finger must be positioned in such a way that pulp-to-pulp contact with the other replanted fingers is possible.

Replanting all the amputated fingers is the first choice in multiple amputations.[41–43] If this is not possible, careful rearrangement of the parts is

important to get the best outcome.[31] When all of the fingers are amputated, and not all of the amputated parts are fit for replantation, preferentially the authors start from the ulnar side.[39] This method will give good grip and a wide web space. During skeletal fixation, adequate care has to be exercised to fix in the right orientation so that rotational deformity problems do not occur. Nothing is more disappointing than to have a surviving thumb and fingers that do not meet.[34]

Fingers do not contain muscle and so can stand long periods of ischemia.[44-46] In spite of this, at all times the amputated parts have to be kept well preserved in cold ischemia and not left to dry or remain at room temperature. At the end of preparation, the parts are replaced into the cold chamber. The fact that they can stand ischemia for long can be used to push the bar of reconstruction including serial replantation as in this case, in which the little finger tip was replanted onto the replanted segment of the middle finger. The pressure head in the digital vessels is quite high, and this makes the second replant in a finger possible.

BILATERAL EXTENSIVE AMPUTATIONS

A 44-year-old man sustained injuries to both hands in a train accident. On the right, he was left with the first metacarpal and the base of the proximal phalanx of the thumb and the proximal body of the hand. Because of the loss of the thenar muscles, the first metacarpal was immobile (**Fig. 3**A). The palmar surface of the residual hand and wrist had been skin grafted. The left side retained a thumb, also relatively immobile except for the basal joint and with circumferential skin graft proximal to it. The proximal body of the hand was skin grafted with graft extending well onto the forearm (see **Fig. 3**B). An attempt to provide better skin cover on the left with an anterolateral thigh flap elsewhere had failed. He depended totally on others for even basic activities.

The authors' initial intention was to provide a mobile post to meet the stable first metacarpal on each side using toe transfers. Because the radial posts were totally fixed, fine pinch was not a goal; it was expected that special appliances attached to small objects, such as pens and pencils, would be required to facilitate hand use, much are routine to the severely disabled rheumatoid hand.

The patient preferred that reconstruction of the right hand be carried out first. The grafted area at the base of the right thumb was excised and replaced with a pedicled groin flap (see **Fig. 3**C). For toe transfer to this hand, the authors prefer the second toe from the left foot for convenience of the lie of the vessels. On dissection of the foot, the authors found that there were no significant veins on the dorsum of the foot as most were thrombosed segmentally, so further dissection had to be abandoned. Retrospectively, the authors realized that, having suffered a bilateral upper limb injury and, later, had multiple surgical procedures, including an attempted free flap, the

dorsal veins of his feet had been used repeatedly for intravenous access, leading to thrombosis of these vessels. The authors then dissected the second toe from the right foot and transferred it successfully to the right hand (see **Fig. 3**D). In such cases, when there has been extensive injury, one should expect the recipient vessels and tendons to be very proximal and be aware that vein and tendon grafts may be needed. He was rehabilitated to provide this hand with pinch and weak grasp functions.

Left side reconstruction also required preliminary groin flap cover of the base of the thumb and remnant of the palm. At this operation, an attempt was made to separate the first and second metacarpals to gain a little mobility of the first ray (see **Fig. 3**E). This hand also needed construction of an ulnar post. Having used the only possible toe transfer, this option no longer existed. The alternative was a bone graft with flap cover. Provision of at least 15 cm of nonvascularized bone graft to meet the thumb tip meet would have been difficult and, also, prone to both resorption and fracture. Providing that length of thin, tubed flap to cover the bone would also have been difficult in a bulky individual. Therefore, a free fibula of 15 cm length was harvested with a large skin island and the flexor hallucis longus muscle (see **Fig. 3**F). The fibula was attached to the carpus in such a position that the thumb could move at its basal joint to meet it. The skin surface pointed to the thumb, and excess skin was draped over the distal end of the bone. The flexor hallucis longus muscle on the noncontact surface was skin grafted. The free fibula flap survived, although there was a nonunion at the proximal contact surface that required secondary iliac bone grafting to achieve union. The patient is now able to pinch and hold objects between the thumb and the free fibula and use it as a good supporting post when using the right hand to manipulate objects (see **Fig. 3**G, H).

Discussion

This presentation illustrates a series of steps that transformed a totally crippling deformity to independence for this individual in respect of activities of daily living and a useful life.

First is to try to plan the whole process from debridement to the ultimate reconstruction.[14,47] When such planning is made, the authors can help by preserving much that will be useful later. For example, avoiding the dorsum of the foot for venous access in major injuries and as a source of vein grafts will help preserve the reconstructive option of toe transfer later. Two mobile digits on

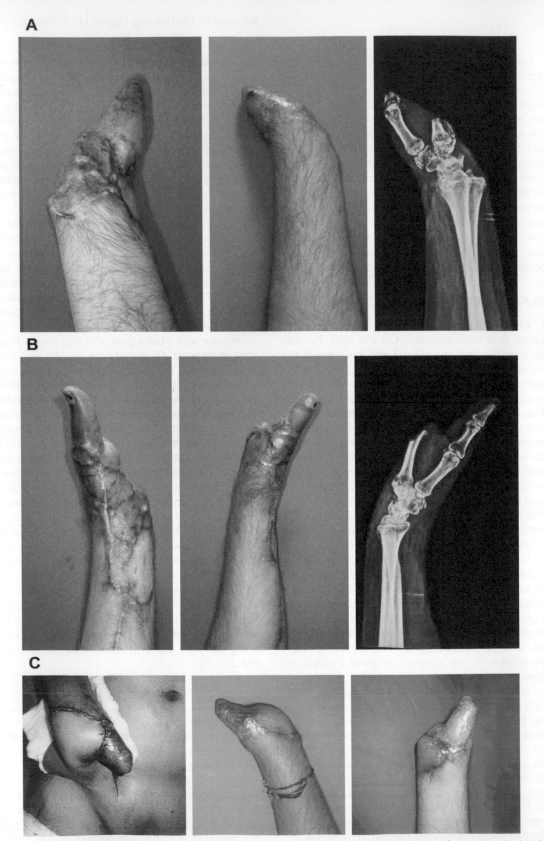

Fig. 3. (*A*) The right hand with just the first metacarpal, with loss of thenar muscles and skin grafted volar side. (*B*) The left hand with immobile thumb with circumferential skin grafted area proximally. The skin graft extends proximally in the forearm, and the linear extension was made for gaining access during the previous unsuccessful attempt at a free flap for cover. (*C*) The right hand is resurfaced with a groin flap to provide a base for the toe transfer.

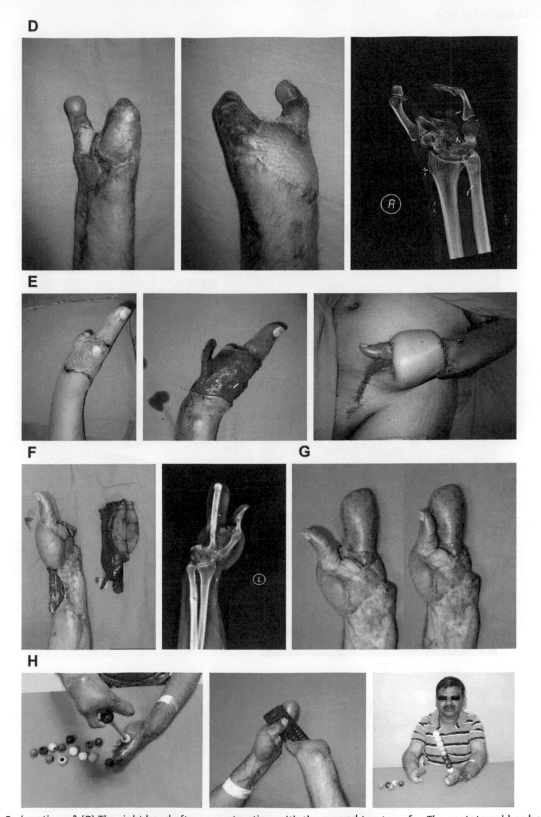

Fig. 3. (*continued*) (*D*) The right hand after reconstruction with the second toe transfer. The metatarsal has been fixed to the carpal bones. (*E*) The left hand is resurfaced with a groin flap after excising the skin-grafted area. The second metacarpal is osteotomized to create a web space. (*F*) The left hand reconstructed by fixing the harvested free fibula on the metacarpal. The skin surface is placed on the contact side and the muscle is skin grafted. The pedicle was extended by vein grafts. (*G*) Images show the functioning of the hand by closing of the thumb to the stable fibular graft. It has developed good lateral pinch power. (*H*) Bimanual activities possible by using one hand for holding and manipulating with the other hand.

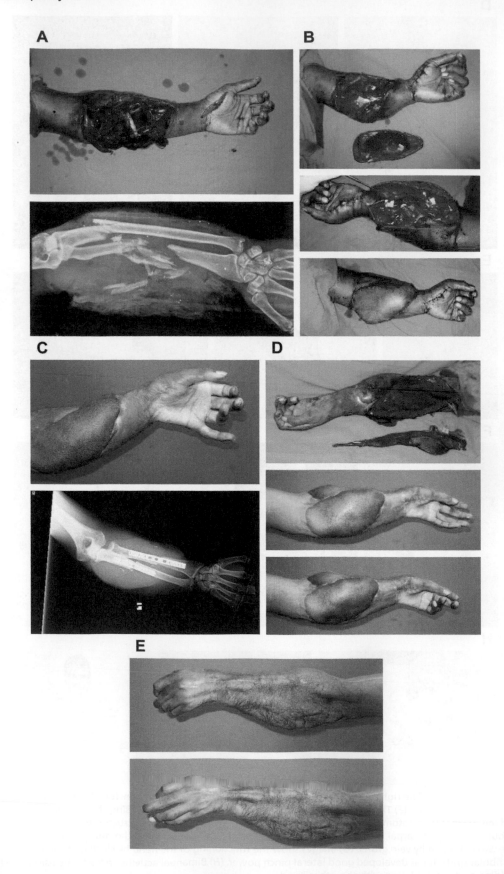

this left hand would have created a much more useful hand.[25]

Whenever an entire thumb or ulnar post is reconstructed by toe transfer from the base, the toe has to be harvested with the metatarsal. The second toe is the only option because taking the great toe with the metatarsal creates too much disability in the donor foot. The metatarsal is bare and without skin cover, so adequate soft tissue cover is always needed. Almost always, a preliminary flap will be needed to provide this.[27] The authors routinely use a pedicled groin flap for this purpose. This flap must be planned such that it can cover the entire length of the pedicle of the toe transfer to the vessel to which it will be anastomosed, so the pedicle can be tunneled comfortably.

When toe transfer is not possible, a stable post can be created in one stage using a free fibular flap, as illustrated earlier. A long skin island and harvest of vascularized flexor hallucis longus in the flap allow complete bone cover, also in a single stage. Being vascularized, graft survival and bone union are more likely. This mode of reconstruction was originally reported by Yildirim and colleagues[48] for management of a 4-limb train accident.

The ultimate usefulness of the hand depends on the ability of the segments of the reconstructed hand to meet.[27] For this, positioning of the imported ray is very important. It is not necessary to achieve anatomically correct positioning. Directional positioning is the need, such that movement of any moving segments is in the direction of the other segments. Mistakes that only achieve scissoring of the segments are not useful.

The space between the reconstructed segments is important because this will determine the size of the objects that can be held. Web space deepening and thinning of flaps may need to be done. However, in a major injury, this has to be done with care, because division of the adductors will result in decrease of pinching force: so, a balance has to be achieved.

AVASCULAR HAND WITH EXTENSIVE SOFT TISSUE LOSS IN THE FOREARM

A 42-year-old man sustained injury in a major road traffic accident resulting in extensive soft tissue loss in the forearm with comminuted segmental fractures of the radius and ulna and loss of the flexor muscles, nerves, and the extensor tendons (**Fig. 4**A). This distal part of the limb was devascularized. Although there was loss of all the external functional components of the hand, the authors planned to salvage the hand because it was structurally intact.[49] Management of this patient required application of all of the principles of reconstruction starting with radical debridement, including excision of all free bone fragments without soft tissue attachment. The forearm bone ends were further shortened to allow primary fixation. After debridement, there was a 6-cm gap in the radial artery and a long proximal loss of the ulnar artery. Distal revascularization was achieved by anastomosing the proximal radial artery to the distal ulnar artery. Shortening of the forearm allowed the authors to achieve a mass repair of the flexor muscles. It also facilitated direct repair of the median and ulnar nerves. Soft tissue cover was achieved with an anterolateral thigh flap, which was anastomosed to the proximal ulnar artery. The distal end of the flap vessel was anastomosed to the distal radial artery (see **Fig. 4**B, C). In this way, the hand was revascularized by inputs from both the ulnar and radial arteries.[50] The wound healed primarily; when some flexor function returned, restoration of wrist and finger extension was carried out using a free functioning gracilis muscle transfer. Proximally, the gracilis was attached to the lateral epicondyle and distally to the extensors of the fingers. The artery was anastomosed end to side to the brachial artery, and a good fascicle of the median nerve was used to motor the muscle. At 1 year after injury, he has a good functioning hand and is able to carry out most basic day-to-day activities (see **Fig. 4**D, E).

Discussion

Road traffic accidents and industrial injuries can result in segmental losses of skin and soft tissues, tendons, and nerves in association with open fractures and distal revascularization. It is the authors' philosophy to salvage these upper limbs if the

Fig. 4. (A) Major crush injury to the left forearm with circumferential degloving injury with skin loss, and radiograph showing the extent of the skeletal injury. (B) The forearm after shortening and fixation and revascularization by direct repair of proximal radial to distal ulnar artery. The anterolateral thigh flap has been revascularized with the ulnar artery, and the distal end is attached to the distal radial artery and the soft tissue cover achieved. (C) The forearm with a well-settled flap and primary bone union. (D, E) Free functioning gracilis muscle transfer to achieve active extension of wrist and fingers.

hand is structurally intact and reconstruction is technically possible.[13,16] This philosophy is based on their experience that, in such cases, even if all of the longitudinal structures have been damaged, or have suffered segmental loss, the hand can be made functional by secondary procedures of the kind described earlier and such a limb will serve patients better than the best available prosthesis at this time. As explained earlier, such cases need a well worked out plan of management, in place from the start, if a good outcome is to be achieved.

Many complex injuries that need revascularization also have severely comminuted fractures and/or bone ends bereft of periosteum. They may also have segmental loss of blood vessels and nerves. It is the authors' practice to shorten the bone to facilitate direct approximation of the blood vessels.[49] This practice saves time by avoiding time-consuming and complex bone fixation techniques in the presence of bone loss. Primary bone union and stability are more likely. Time wasting at the bone fixation stage has to be avoided to reduce ischemia time, as bone fixation must precede revascularization, except in exceptional circumstances, when a temporary arterial shunt is used. Although the muscle mass distally may be less, a short ischemia time is vital for recovery of intrinsic muscle function. Shortening also avoids the need for vein grafts and, sometimes, nerve grafts, also reducing the total surgical time.

Although the authors used a flow through flap for cover in this case, these constitute less than 2% of all such cases requiring revascularisation in their experience. This rarity is because the geometry and pattern of deficit of the vessels and the soft tissue are so variable that it is difficult to plan and achieve such a composite reconstruction. Time may be wasted in planning, which cannot be afforded in the presence of distal devascularization. Further, if there is any problem with the proximal anastomosis of the flap, both the flap and the distal part will undergo necrosis. The authors preferred option is to use a vein graft to revascularize the distal segment and then cover the area with a flap vascularized independently of the artery supplying the distal part.

In total compartment loss, it is necessary to replace at least some musculotendinous functions. This replacement may be achieved by secondary repair with tendon grafts or tendon transfers, with or without selective arthrodeses. In long segmental losses whereby the proximal end is in the muscular area, secondary repair with grafts is not possible. When the other compartment is also injured, tendon transfers

are also not possible. In such cases, if flexor power is weak, use of the hand can be enhanced by tenodesis of the flexor tendons at the wrist. It is also worthwhile to add some power to the extensor side. This can be done with the use of free functioning muscle transfers, and gracilis is the muscle commonly used.[51–53] The muscle is attached well proximally in the arm, revascularized by end to side anastomosis to the brachial artery, and motored by suture of the gracilis motor nerve to a good fascicle of the median nerve. A vital requirement is that the route of passage of the free functioning muscle transfer has to have good soft tissue cover. One also needs to wait for the induration following the injury and primary surgery to subside. Another significant factor is that the ischemia time during transfer is kept as short as possible when the muscle is to be used for function, and the authors strive to keep this to less than 1.5 hours. This time is in contrast to than when using free muscle flaps for soft tissue cover only, when the ischemia time can be longer.

AVASCULAR HAND WITH INJURY IN THE PROXIMAL PART OF THE HAND

A 63-year-old man sustained a crush avulsion injury of the hand and forearm (**Fig. 5**A). The injury included avulsion of the vessels in the palm, leaving the fingers devascularized. Debridement included the little finger, leaving a need to revascularize the index, middle, and ring fingers. A vein graft was harvested from the dorsum of the foot with 2 venous limbs proximally. After reversal of the vein, each proximal limb was used to anastomose a common digital artery (see **Fig. 5**B). The critical raw area over the grafts was reconstructed with an anterolateral thigh flap (see **Fig. 5**C). The patient made a good functional recovery (see **Fig. 5**D).

Discussion

Vein grafts are the easiest and quickest way to bridge defects in vessels. The vessel ends are trimmed to good and healthy segments before anastomosis. When multiple segments are to be revascularized distally, harvesting vein grafts with a branching pattern to match the defect, such as in the case earlier, are useful and save time. Veins of the lower limb are thicker than the veins of the upper limb. When vein grafts from the leg are used for upper limb reconstruction, they are predilated with saline after harvest to reduce spasm after repair. This whole raw area is covered with anterolateral thigh flap. In this way, good functional outcome is achieved.

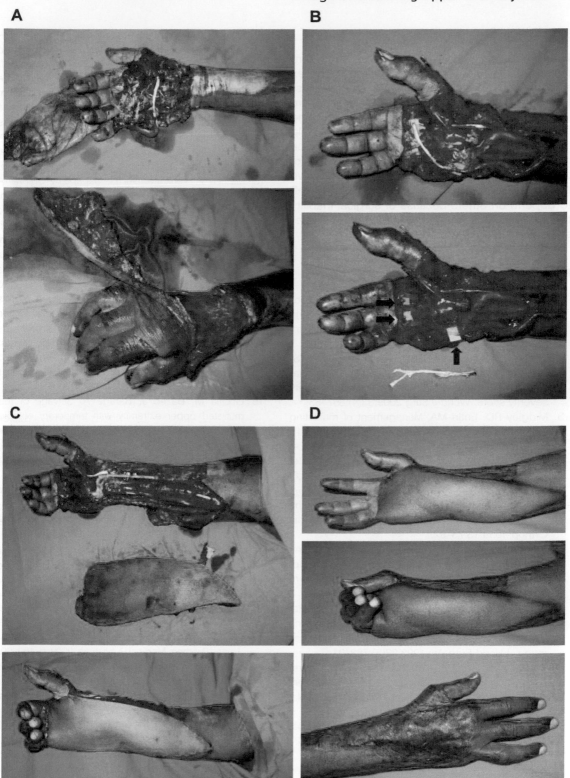

Fig. 5. (*A*) Crush avulsion injury of the hand and forearm with devascularized fingers. (*B*) Postdebridement picture with the thumb positioned in abducted position. The yellow background strips (*arrows*) show the location of the ulnar artery and the common digital vessels. The harvested vein graft by the side of the hand for revascularization of both the common digital arteries. (*C*) The raw area covered with anterolateral thigh flap attached to the radial artery. (*D*) Postoperative result at 1 year.

SUMMARY

These cases underscore several important principles of management of these complex surgical problems. Perhaps, above all, they illustrate the philosophy that all but the most severe injuries with no functional components remaining of the hand itself are beyond reconstructive help and that basic function can almost always be restored by surgeons with a complete plastic, orthopedic, and hand surgical reconstructive armamentarium. Few persons should ever be left to depend on others because of surgical inability to perform this surgery or unwillingness to refer such individuals to those who can.

REFERENCES

1. Togawa S, Yamami N, Nakayama H, et al. The validity of the mangled extremity severity score in the assessment of upper limb injuries. J Bone Joint Surg Br 2005;87(11):1516–9.
2. Prichayudh S, Verananvattna A, Sriussadaporn S, et al. Management of upper extremity vascular injury: outcome related to the mangled extremity severity score. World J Surg 2009;33(4):857–63.
3. Midgley RD, Entin MA. Management of mutilating injuries of the hand. Clin Plast Surg 1976;3(1): 99–109.
4. Brown HC, William HB, Woodhouse FM. Principles of salvage in mutilating hand injuries. J Trauma 1968;8: 319–32.
5. McCormack RM. Reconstructive surgery and the immediate care of the severely injured hand. Clin Orthop 1959;13:75–82.
6. Stanger K, Horch RE, Dragu A. Severe mutilating injuries with complex macroamputations of the upper extremity - is it worth the effort? World J Emerg Surg 2015;10:30.
7. Graham B, Adkins P, Tsai TM, et al. Major replantation versus revision amputation and prosthetic fitting in the upper extremity: a late functional outcomes study. J Hand Surg Am 1998;23(5):783–91.
8. Peacock K, Tsai TM. Comparison of functional results of replantation versus prosthesis in a patient with bilateral arm amputation. Clin Orthop Relat Res 1987;(214):153–9.
9. O'Keeffe B. Prosthetic rehabilitation of the upper limb amputee. Indian J Plast Surg 2011;44(2): 246–52.
10. Bertrand AA, Sen S, Otake LR, et al. Changing attitudes toward hand allotransplantation among North American hand surgeons. Ann Plast Surg 2014;72(Suppl 1):S56–60.
11. Alolabi N, Chuback J, Grad S, et al. The utility of hand transplantation in hand amputee patients. J Hand Surg Am 2015;40(1):8–14.
12. Dias JJ, Chung KC, Garcia-Elias M, et al. Recommendations for the improvement of hand injury care across the world. Injury 2006;37(11):1078–82.
13. Sabapathy SR, Bhardwaj P. Microsurgery and complex hand injuries. In: Cheema TA, editor. Complex injuries of the hand. London: JP Medical Publishers; 2014. p. 233–54.
14. Sabapathy SR, Venkatramani H. Massive upper limb trauma. In: Trail IA, Fleming ANM, editors. Disorder of the hand. London: Springer; 2015. p. 391–414.
15. Mathew P, Venkatramani H, Sabapathy SR. Miniabdominal flaps for preservation of digital length in an 18-month old child. J Hand Surg Eur Vol 2013; 38(1):89–91.
16. Sabapathy SR. Amputations and replantations. In: Chung KC, Disa JJ, Gosain AK, et al, editors. Plastic surgery – indications and practice. New York: Elsevier; 2009. p. 1211–24.
17. Atkins SE, Winterton RIS, Kay SP. Upper limb amputations: where, when and how to replant. Curr Orthop 2008;22:31–41.
18. Kokkoli E, Spyropoulou GA, Shih HS, et al. Heterotopic procedures in mutilating hand injuries: a synopsis of essential reconstructive tools. Plast Reconstr Surg 2015;136(5):1015–26.
19. Godina M, Bazec J, Baraga A. Salvage of the mutilated upper extremity with temporary ectopic implantation of the undamaged part. Plast Reconstr Surg 1986;78(3):295–9.
20. Brown RE, Wu TY. Use of "spare parts" in mutilated upper extremity injuries. Hand Clin 2003;19(1):73–87.
21. Gupta A, Shatford RA, Wolff TW, et al. Instructional course lectures, the American Academy of Orthopaedic Surgeons - treatment of the severely injured upper extremity. J Bone Joint Surg Am 1999;81(11): 1628–51.
22. Lister G, Scheker LR. Emergency free flaps to the upper extremity. J Hand Surg Am 1988;13:22–8.
23. Sabapathy SR, Rajasekaran S. Management of complex injuries of the upper extremity proximal to the wrist. In: Venkataswami R, editor. Surgery of the injured hand – towards functional restoration. Delhi: Jaypee Brothers Medical Publishers; 2009. p. 150–60.
24. Littler JW. On making a thumb: one hundred years of surgical effort. J Hand Surg Am 1976,1(1):35–51.
25. Moran SL, Berger RA. Biomechanics and hand trauma: what you need. Hand Clin 2003;19(1):17–31.
26. Lees VC, Wren C, Elliot D. Internal splints for prevention of first web contracture following severe disruption of the first web space. J Hand Surg Br 1994;19:560–2.
27. Sabapathy SR, Venkatramani H, Bhardwaj P. Reconstruction of the thumb amputation at the carpometacarpal joint level by groin flap and second toe transfer. Injury 2013;44(3):370–5.
28. Sabapathy SR, Bajantri B. Indications, selection, and use of distant pedicled flap for upper limb reconstruction. Hand Clin 2014;30(2):185–99.

29. Bajantri B, Latheef L, Sabapathy SR. Tips to orient pedicled groin flap for hand defects. Tech Hand Up Extrem Surg 2013;17(2):68–71.

30. Sabapathy SR, Satbhai NG. Microsurgery in the urgent and emergent management of the hand. Curr Rev Musculoskelet Med 2014;7(1):40–6.

31. Sabapathy SR, Venkatramani H, Bharathi RR, et al. Replantation surgery. J Hand Surg Am 2011;36(6): 1104–10.

32. Sabapathy SR. Replantation. Semin Plast Surg 2013;27(4):163–4.

33. Sabapathy SR, Bhardwaj P. Secondary procedures in replantation. Semin Plast Surg 2013;27(4):198–204.

34. Venkatramani H, Bhardwaj P, Sierakowski A, et al. Functional outcomes of post-traumatic metacarpal hand reconstruction with free toe-to-hand transfer. Indian J Plast Surg 2016;49(1):16–25.

35. Wei FC. Tissue preservation in hand injury: the first step to toe-to-hand transplantation [editorial]. Plast Reconstr Surg 1998;102:2497–501.

36. Yim KK, Wei FC. Secondary procedures to improve function after to-to-hand transfers. Br J Plast Surg 1995;48:487–91.

37. Morrison WA, McCombe D. Digital replantation. Hand Clin 2007;23(1):1–12.

38. Solarz MK, Thoder JJ, Rehman S. Management of major traumatic upper extremity amputations. Orthop Clin North Am 2016;47(1):127–36.

39. Elliot D, Henley M, Sammut D. Selective replantation with ulnar translocation in multidigital amputations. Br J Plast Surg 1994;47:318–23.

40. del Piñal F. Severe mutilating injuries to the hand: guidelines for organizing the chaos. J Plast Reconstr Aesthet Surg 2007;60(7):816–27.

41. Cong H, Sui H, Wang C, et al. Ten-digit replantation with seven years follow-up: a case report. Microsurgery 2010;30(5):405–9.

42. Kwon GD, Ahn BM, Lee JS, et al. Clinical outcomes of a simultaneous replantation technique for amputations of four or five digits. Microsurgery 2016; 36(3):225–9.

43. Woo SH, Cheon HJ, Kim YW, et al. Delayed and suspended replantation for complete amputation of digits and hands. J Hand Surg Am 2015;40(5):883–9.

44. Rose EH, Norris MS, Kowalski TA. Microsurgical management of complex fingertip injuries: comparison to conventional skin grafting. J Reconstr Microsurg 1988;4(2):89–98.

45. Venkatramani H, Sabapathy SR. Fingertip replantation: technical considerations and outcome analysis of 24 consecutive fingertip replantations. Indian J Plast Surg 2011;44(2):237–45.

46. Wei FC, Chang YL, Chen HC, et al. Three successful digital replantations in a patient after 84, 86, and 94 hours of cold ischemia time. Plast Reconstr Surg 1998;82(2):346–50.

47. Sabapathy SR, Soucacos PN. Recent advances in trauma and reconstructive surgery of the hand and upper extremity. Guest editorial. Injury 2013;44(3): 281–2.

48. Yildirim S, Akan M, Aköz T. Toe-to-hand transfer from a cross-foot replantation in a traumatic four-extremity amputation. J Reconstr Microsurg 2005;21(7):453–8.

49. Sabapathy SR, Venkatramani H, Bharathi RR, et al. Technical considerations and functional outcome of 22 major replantations (The BSSH Douglas Lamb Lecture, 2005). J Hand Surg Eur Vol 2007;32(5): 488–501.

50. Qing L, Wu P, Liang J, et al. Use of flow through anterolateral thigh perforator flaps in reconstruction of complex extremity defects. J Reconstr Microsurg 2015;31(8):571–8.

51. Oishi SN, Ezaki M. Free gracilis transfer to restore finger flexion in Volkmann ischemic contracture. Tech Hand Up Extrem Surg 2010;14(2):104–7.

52. Sabapathy SR, Elliot D. Complex injuries to the flexors in the hand and forearm. In: Cheema TA, editor. Complex injuries of the hand. London: JP Medical Publishers; 2014. p. 115–28.

53. Venkatramani H, Bhardwaj P. Volkmann's ischemic contracture. In: Chung KC, editor. Essentials of hand surgery. London: JP Medical Limited; 2015. p. 331–48.

Index

Note: Page numbers of article titles are in **boldface** type.

Hand Clin 32 (2016) 599–602
http://dx.doi.org/10.1016/S0749-0712(16)30096-8
0749-0712/16/$ – see front matter

Printed and bound by CPI Group (UK) Ltd, Croydon, CR0 4YY

03/10/2024

01040302-0016